The Anatomists' Library

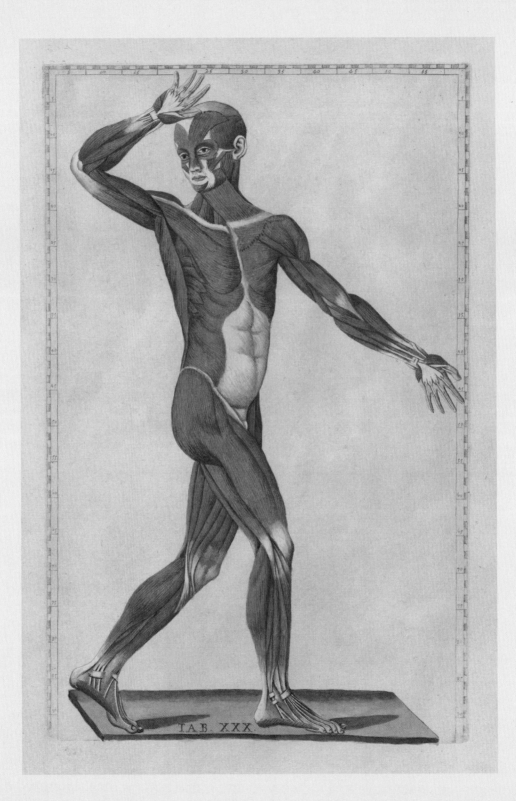

TAB. XXX.

The Anatomists' Library

The Books that Unlocked the Secrets of the Human Body

COLIN SALTER

IVY PRESS

First published in the UK in 2023 by
Ivy Press
An imprint of The Quarto Group
One Triptych Place, London,
United Kingdom, SE1 9SH
T (0)20 7700 6700
www.Quarto.com

British Library Cataloguing-in-Publication Data
A catalogue record for this book is available
from the British Library.

ISBN 978-0-7112-8074-8
eBook ISBN 978-0-7112-8076-2

Printed in China

10 9 8 7 6 5 4 3 2 1

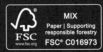

MIX
Paper | Supporting
responsible forestry
FSC® C016973
FSC
www.fsc.org

CONTENTS

INTRODUCTION

B ooks are time capsules. They preserve the knowledge and the attitudes of their age. This is true of all books, even of science fiction, which may conjure extraordinarily inventive futures or pasts, but only from the perspective of the present in which it was written. Writers cannot imagine the unimaginable. This is especially true of non-fiction, which records the truth as it was understood at the time of writing. Knowledge expands, cultures evolve, and successive books on any subject demonstrate these changes. Put them all in a single library and they combine to present a social and scientific history of the wisdom in question.

Anatomy can make a strong case for being the oldest science, with a written history stretching back thousands of years. The anatomist's library, presented in these chapters, contains a fraction of the published works of anatomy, but nevertheless covers well over 150 books spanning more than 5,000 years – from the Edwin Smith Papyrus, which describes the surgical treatment of combat injuries in ancient Egypt, to the current edition of *Musculoskeletal MRI*, reflecting technological advances in the twenty-first century, and *The Human Anatomy and Physiology Coloring Book*, a book for children that shows just how far society has come in overcoming the myth and mistrust which surrounded anatomy for so long.

It's only natural that anatomy should have preoccupied humanity for so long. Our bodies are our selves. Whether or not we believe that they contain our souls, they

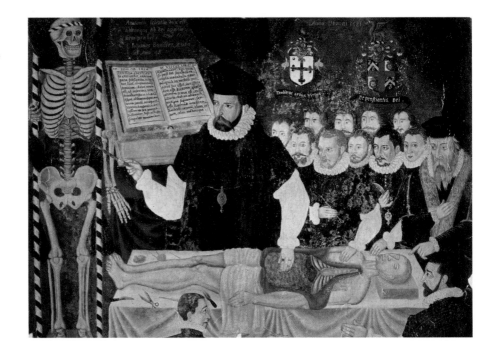

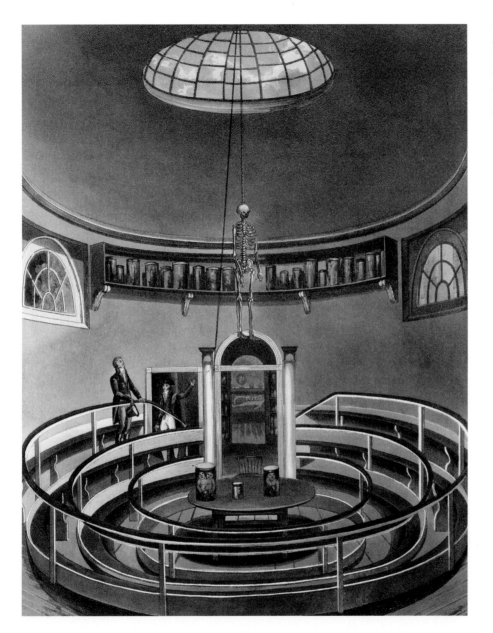

LEFT

Anatomy theatre at the University of Cambridge (1815)

A skeleton suspended over the dissecting table was a *memento mori* as much as a teaching aid.

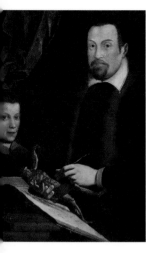

certainly hold our blood and our beating hearts, our lives and (one way or another) our mortality. The American comedian Allan Sherman, in his brilliant anatomical parody of the song 'You Gotta Have Heart', sang:

Skin is what you feel at home in
And without it, furthermore,
Both your liver and abdomen
Would keep falling on the floor.

'Looking in detail at human anatomy,' Alice Roberts, the popular British medical writer and broadcaster, has said, 'I'm always left with two practically irreconcilable thoughts: our bodies are wonderful, intricate masterpieces; and then they are cobbled-together, rag-bag, sometimes clunking machines.' They are extraordinary self-regulating, self-repairing machines; but when they break down or leak, often through the brutality or carelessness of our fellow human beings or ourselves, we want to be able to fix them.

If the earliest application of anatomy was on the battlefield, it soon took on a more spiritual aspect. With the development of philosophical ideas (as explored in this book's sister publication *The Philosopher's Library*) by ancient thinkers in Egypt and Greece, the concept of a soul was born. Soul and thought, detached from the practical functions of the body, were nevertheless held to be contained within it. Early anatomists engaged in furious academic debate about the relative roles of the head and the heart. Where did the soul reside? Which was the seat of reason? In an anatomical hierarchy, did the heart rule the head, or vice versa? We are, in a more metaphorical way, having the same arguments today, when we ask ourselves, 'Do I follow my head, or my heart?'

Anatomy is not immune to global events. Wars between civilisations drove early curiosity about the body. Later, when the Roman Empire collapsed in the fifth century, ushering in a period of barbarism in western Europe, new centres of learning sprung up to the east, launching an Islamic Golden Age which made significant contributions to the study of anatomy. And at the end of that age, western scholars visited the former centres of Islamic learning in Spain to translate Islamic texts back into Latin. In the twentieth century, the horrors of the Second World War contributed to the publication of what many consider the finest anatomical illustrations ever. The four-volume *Topographic Anatomy of Man* by Austrian anatomist Eduard Pernkopf cannot, however, be seen in isolation; it is forever tainted by its association with the atrocities committed by the Nazis in the conflict.

Through experimental dissection, early anatomists such as Herophilos, Galen, Rhazes and Avicenna began to explore the truth about what goes on beneath the skin, and to record their findings in books. Myths were dispelled or perpetuated – for example, that the veins carried blood produced in the liver and the arteries were ducts for a mystical energy called pneuma, which was inhaled along with the air we breathe, stoking the imagined fires of life.

If the world was made of air, earth, fire and water, natural philosophers argued, then the body must be composed of comparable materials – black bile, yellow bile, blood and phlegm. An imbalance of these so-called 'humors' must then be responsible for illnesses of the body. The theory of humorism, of which Galen was a leading proponent, persisted in anatomy literature for centuries, even after the reality of the circulation of blood was discovered by William Harvey in the seventeenth century. Doctors would, it was said, 'rather err with Galen than proclaim the truth with Harvey.'

It was a brave and difficult step for any anatomist to dissociate himself from the prevailing influence of religion on anatomical theory. The Catholic Church had a powerful grip on society in the Middle Ages and one unfortunate Spanish anatomist, Miguel Servet, was burnt alive on a pyre of his books for daring to challenge its orthodoxy. Gradually however, science began to separate from church and state.

That liberation gave anatomists the opportunity to explore the human body purely for the sake of knowledge. The modern science of anatomy was born in the sixteenth century,

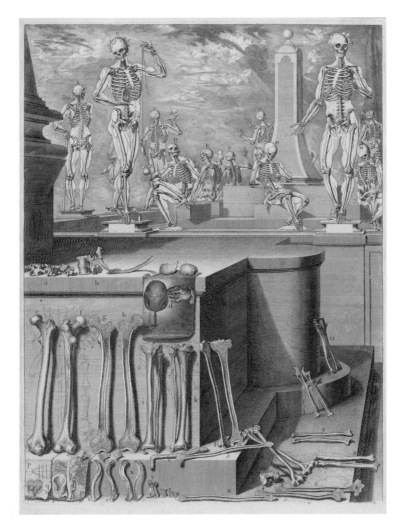

LEFT
Fourteen Skeletons (*c.*1740)

Life and death, in an eighteenth-century engraving after Crisóstomo Martínez (1628–94).

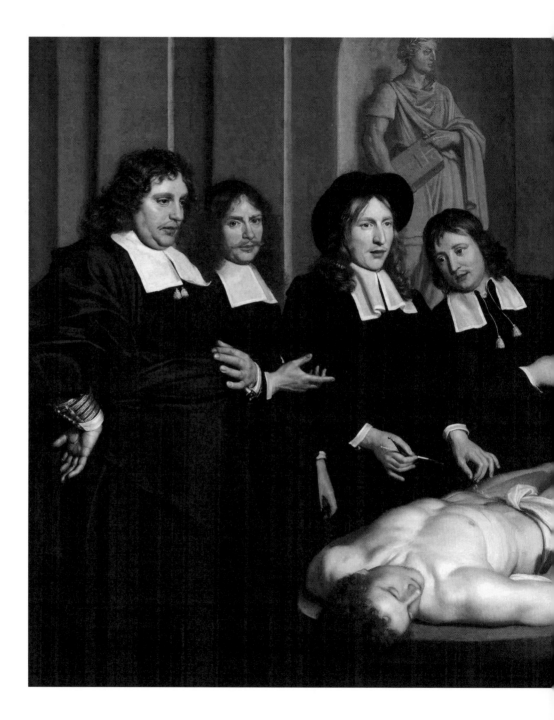

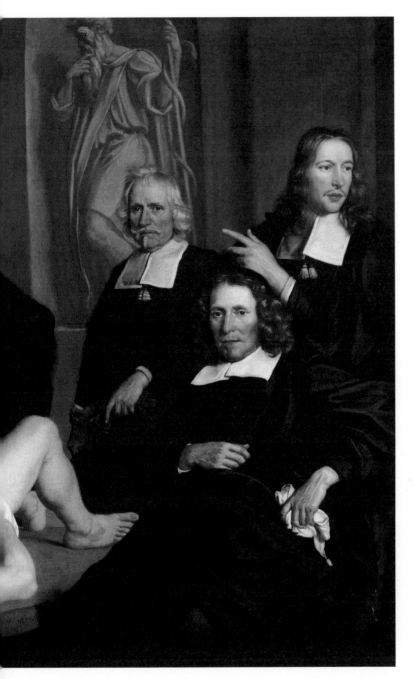

LEFT

The Anatomy Lesson of
Dr Frederik Ruysch (1670)

Ruysch (1638–1731), painted
by Dutch artist Adriaen Backer
(1635–84), developed an
early technique for preserving
human tissue.

initially swept along by the thirst for truth of the Italian Renaissance. It wasn't only surgeons who needed to understand the body; sculptors and painters also wanted to be able to depict the human form to perfection. Artists started to attend public demonstrations of anatomy, and even to learn how to dissect corpses themselves. The spaces between the bookshelves in the anatomist's library are decorated with astonishing examples of artists' understanding of the body.

The supply of bodies for dissection has been a challenge and a source of controversy throughout the history of anatomy. Social conventions have often made any dissection illegal, blasphemous or at least distasteful. At other times it was considered an additional punishment that criminals executed for their crimes would be dissected after death. In London the Barber-Surgeons' Hall was deliberately built on a site near Newgate Prison, from which a steady supply of bodies could be expected. As the popularity of anatomy courses increased from the seventeenth to the nineteenth century, supply could not keep up with demand, and body snatchers stole freshly buried corpses and sold them to needy lecturers and students. This book includes the sensational account of the trial of two such graverobbers in Edinburgh in 1829, and a notebook bound with the skin of one of them. Leonardo da Vinci and Michelangelo both had back-door arrangements with local hospitals to get access to fresh cadavers for the purpose of study.

Anatomy has been taught in art schools ever since the Renaissance. Animator Walt Disney attended drawing classes ten years before he launched his first character, Mickey Mouse, in 1928. Later he recalled, 'Our most difficult job was to develop the cartoon's unnatural but seemingly natural anatomy for humans and animals.' Understanding anatomy was as important to Disney as it was to Albrecht Dürer, the great sixteenth-century illustrator, who famously produced a quite anatomically accurate image of a rhinoceros without ever having seen one. Dürer produced one of the earliest anatomy books for artists rather than surgeons.

The relationship between art and anatomy is a symbiotic one, and illustrations in anatomy books over the ages tell as good a story as the text itself. From the frog-like, whole-figure diagrams of some early Islamic texts, to focussed and accurate drawings of specific organs, anatomy has adopted the latest visual technology to present itself from age to age. It was an early adopter of printing when many books were still copied by hand. For example, *The Wounded Man* – the unfortunate figure designed to exhibit as

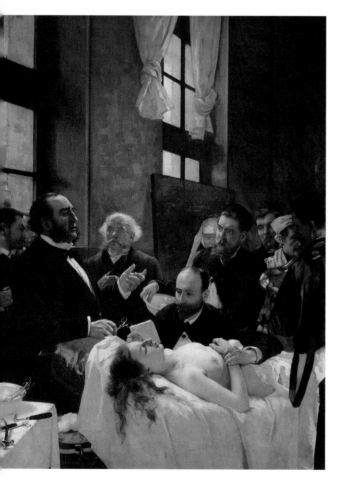

BELOW
Before the Operation (1889)

Jules-Émile Péan (1830–98) was one of the finest French surgeons of his day, shown here with his students in a painting by Henri Gervex (1852–1929).

many different types of injury in a single image as possible – was illustrated with crude woodblocks. Woodcarving skills became more refined through the medieval period before giving way to the fine detail made possible by lithography in the Renaissance. The invention of photography made greater realism possible, although often an idealised image by an artist was better than a photograph at showing the intended details, especially with the refinement of colour printing in the nineteenth century.

The technological advances in how we look at anatomy – from the invention of the microscope in the seventeenth century to that of the endoscope in the early nineteenth, from the discovery of X-rays to the CT and MRI scans of today – have transformed the way in which anatomy can be made visual. Scan images can be artificially coloured to highlight the details they have captured.

In the twenty-first century an anatomical image from an MRI scan is as likely to be an online three-dimensional view as a printed two-dimensional still. Perhaps, in the internet age, the anatomy book will become a thing entirely of the past. This book concentrates on those published up to the end of the nineteenth century. By then, human macroscopic anatomy (the anatomy visible to the naked eye) was more or less complete. There was a name for every part, and a good understanding of how all the parts worked together to keep us alive and moving. From the twentieth century onwards, the great advances in anatomy have been at the cellular or subcellular level, and anatomy is in a new, microscopic phase.

The history of anatomy is the history of how we overcome our physical shortcomings. Another great animator, Chuck Jones, who created some of the world's most recognisable cartoon characters including Bugs Bunny and his nemesis Wile E. Coyote, once commented, 'The Coyote is limited, as Bugs is limited, by his anatomy.' We are all limited by our anatomy. By writing about it and illustrating it, by reading about it and seeing it, we can understand our limitations and sometimes even conquer them. Each of us lives in a marvellous machine, our body: finely tuned and at the same time a delicate chaos of interdependent systems, constantly at risk of failure. To know anatomy is, in a very real sense, to know our selves.

Colin Salter
Edinburgh
September 2022

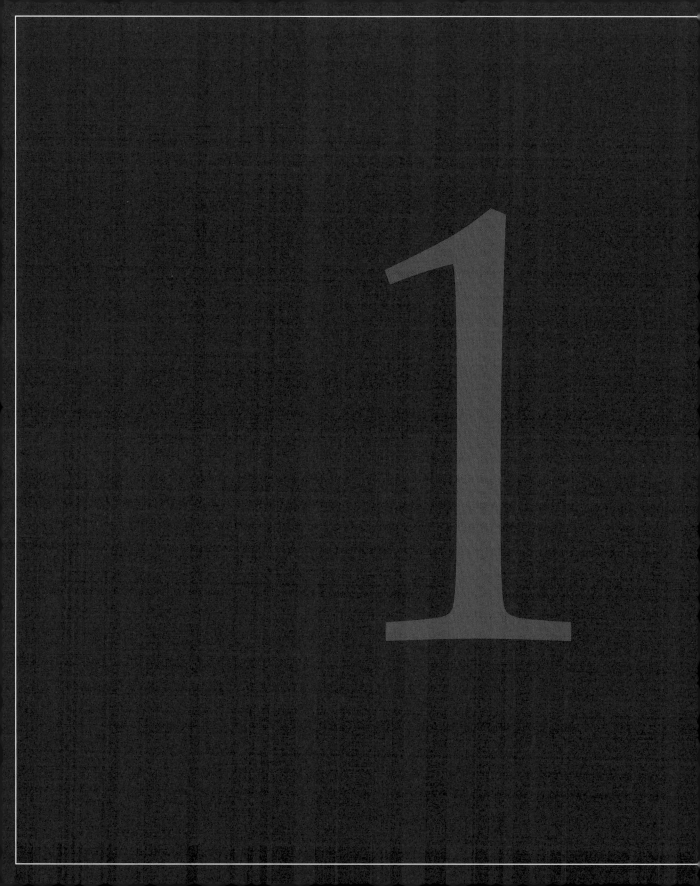

ANATOMY IN THE ANCIENT WORLD

3000 BCE–1300 CE

By the beginning of the fourteenth century, the medical profession had effectively been using the same textbook for 1,300 years. Practitioners still relied on herbal remedies, leeches and the surgeon's saw to cure most ills. Anatomical knowledge remained sketchy and inaccurate, based largely on the dissection of apes and pigs and muddled by religious and philosophical dogma.

The 'textbook' in question was actually a vast body of work by the prolific medical author Claudius Galenus, who lived in the first and second centuries of the Common Era (CE). Galen (to use the modern form of his name) advanced the science of anatomy further than any other person in history. In doing so, however, he built on thousands of years of experimental knowledge of the human body. Modern anatomists and their librarians owe Galen a considerable debt, not only for his own contributions, but for his observations of the thinking – right and wrong – of his ancient predecessors. In many cases, where original documents are long lost, Galen's notes about them are the only record of their ideas.

1 Ancient Egypt

The earliest records of anatomy to survive are Egyptian papyri, themselves about 3,600 years old, but which include copies of earlier documents which may have been written up to 5,000 years ago. One appears to have been a military handbook for the treatment of a variety of injuries including head trauma. It is known today as the Edwin Smith Papyrus, after the American antiquarian who bought it in Luxor in 1862. It is unique among the handful of known medical papyri in being a thoroughly practical manual, with treatments based on observation and practice rather than incantations and superstition – although it does also contain a handful of magic spells as a last resort. It was first translated in 1930 and found to contain the oldest known use of anatomical terminology, including the first appearance of the hieroglyph for the brain (literally 'skull offal'). It describes parts of the brain and the impact of cranial injuries on the rest of the body. Today it is a jewel in the collection of the New York Academy of Medicine.

Severe injury was then, as at many times in the history of anatomy, the only opportunity to see the inside of a living (or dying) human body. The Egyptian tradition of mummification also afforded glimpses of the organs, albeit in a ritual rather than a scientific context; and the skeleton was known from long-dead human remains. Deliberate dissection for mere intellectual curiosity was a violation of the repository of the soul, philosophically and legally out of the question.

Nevertheless, the Edwin Smith Papyrus offers a very modern diagnostic process for spinal injury and a recognition of the relationship between heartbeat and pulse. Another work of comparable age discusses the role of the heart in the circulation of all bodily fluids and therefore in all mental and physical diseases. A German Egyptologist, Georg Ebers, bought it from Edwin Smith in Luxor in 1872, and it now resides in the University of Leipzig, where Ebers was a professor. It contains a great many incantations and spells, but also demonstrates some empirical knowledge of anatomy. There are sections on dentistry, problems of the skin, eyes, intestines and gynaecology (including contraception). 'To prevent conception,' it advises, 'smear a paste of dates, acacia, and honey to wool and apply as a pessary.'

BELOW

Egyptian hieroglyphics

The Egyptians, who were medically advanced, wrote the oldest surviving anatomical texts. These four characters, from *c.*1700 BCE, spell the ancient Egyptian word for the brain.

ABOVE

The Edwin Smith Papyrus
(*c.*3000 BCE)

The earliest known surgical
document describes the
detailed treatment of forty-
eight conditions, many of
them the results of injury
in battle.

The Georg Ebers Papyrus is one of the few ancient texts to exist in two copies – the Carlsberg Papyrus, of later date, is identical to the Ebers. The Brugsch Papyrus, in Berlin, is a different text which covers much of the same ground as the Ebers and Carlsberg items, and from the details within it some historians think Galen himself may have consulted it. The Kahun Papyrus, written in around 1800 BCE and now kept at University College London, also deals with pregnancy, fertility and gynaecological diseases.

The Hearst Papyrus is named after Phoebe Hearst (mother of the tycoon William Randolph Hearst), who led the archaeological expedition during which it was discovered in 1901. It deals with problems of the blood, hair and urine, among other things. One of the conditions it describes is 'the Canaanite illness . . . when the body is coal-black with charcoal spots.' It's believed to be a copy made in around 1800 BCE of an earlier work, although there is currently some doubt about its authenticity.

The brain, as mere skull offal, was not understood and, indeed, not preserved during mummification. Egyptians seem to have had little knowledge of the kidneys, and thought that the heart drove the circulation of all fluids – urine, semen and tears, as well as blood. Together, however, their observations in the various papyri place Egyptian medicine far ahead of the more celebrated Greek schools which dominated the science a thousand years later.

2 Ancient Greece

The rise of Greece as a centre of power and learning prompted a new interest in the natural world. As natural philosophers identified the fundamental elements which made up the physical environment – earth, air, fire, water and others – they turned their attention to the human form and its composition. A shadowy figure, Alcmaeon of Croton (b. *c.*510 BCE), who may have been a student of Pythagoras in the fifth century BCE, was probably among the first to undertake dissections of animals in pursuit of knowledge about human anatomy. Little is known of his life, but he is credited with discovering the optic nerves and the Eustachian tubes, part of the middle ear. He conducted a lot of work on the sensory organs and deduced that they were connected to the brain, which he considered the seat of thought and the soul. The truth of this would be contested for centuries by those who argued that the heart was centre of life; but Alcmaeon was, of course, correct.

Grander claims have been made for Alcmaeon, too – that he was the first to dissect a human cadaver and the first to write an anatomical treatise, *On Nature*. He's even been cited as the author of the first book of animal fables, ahead of Aesop; although a contemporary of his, the Spartan poet Alcman, seems the more likely candidate. Alcman sometimes gets the credit for Alcmaeon's remark that 'experience is the beginning of learning,' but the phrase certainly chimes with Alcmaeon's reputed reliance on empirical anatomical evidence. The need to see for oneself, to trust only the evidence of one's eyes, is a tenet which could be said to underpin every advance in anatomy throughout history; and, conversely, a reliance on the unchallenged views of the past has at many times held science back.

Alcmaeon's greatest claim to fame was a mistake. He was the first to propose the concept of humors, the bodily fluids flowing through our veins which must be in balance to maintain good health. The word 'humor' comes from the Greek word for sap. He was wrong, of course; but chiming as it did with the earth-air-fire-water school of thought, humor theory prevailed for some 2,000 years. Alcmaeon subscribed to a broader palette of humors than later medical theorists. The most familiar to us today are: blood, phlegm, yellow bile and black bile. An excess of any one caused changes in health and mood: one might be sanguine (with too much blood), phlegmatic (from phlegm), choleric (from yellow bile) or melancholic (from the Greek word for black). In Alcmaeon's words, 'the equality of the powers (wet, dry, cold, hot, bitter, sweet, etc.) maintains health but monarchy among them produces disease.'

Neither *On Nature* nor any other of Alcmaeon's writings survive, and no details of his life are known except his birthplace in southern Italy (then part of Greater Greece). Because of this obscuring fog he is often overlooked in histories of anatomy. Nevertheless, what little we do know of

BELOW
Quinta Essentia (1574)

An illustration from Leonhart Thurneisser's book showing the four 'humors', of which the human body was supposed to consist – Flegmatic, Sanguin, Coleric and Melancholy – along with astrological symbols and a half-male, half-female figure.

him is thanks to references in the works of other writers who evidently held him in high regard. He merited a place in *Parallel Lives*, Plutarch's collection of biographies; in the anthologies of Greek scholarship collected by Joannes Stobaeus of Macedonia; in the writings of Greek polymath Theophrastus of Lesbos; and, like so many other lost pioneers, in the works of Galen.

3 The Hippocratic Corpus

Alcmaeon's *On Nature* earns its place in any imaginary anatomist's library, even if no hard copy survives. The author (and his contemporaries Pausanias, Acron and Philistion of Locri) performed the first dissections in pursuit of science and had a profound influence on generations of anatomists including Hippocrates (*c.*460–370 BCE). Working less than a century after Alcmaeon, Hippocrates is revered as the father of medicine, the pioneer in whose name doctors, until recently, took the Hippocratic Oath which defined their code of practice (a more modern code of ethics is now in place). He also played his part in the development of anatomy.

The Hippocratic Oath's best-known line may be the promise, 'I will abstain from all intentional wrong-doing and harm.' But it also includes the assurance, 'I will not use the knife, not even, verily, on sufferers from stone, but I will give place to such as are craftsmen therein.' This suggests that there was already a distinction between doctors and surgeons, and a mutual respect. Hippocrates developed systems of medical examination by hand, eye and ear which are still used today; and although he left incision to others, he maintained that a working knowledge of anatomy was essential for good doctoral practice, describing it as 'the basis of medical discourse.'

Beyond the medical ethics and patient assessment techniques which he bequeathed, Hippocrates' greatest gift to all branches of medicine may be his insistence on separating health from religion. His family were priests on the Greek island of Kos and through them he inherited his right to practice medicine. Like many sons, however, he refused to follow in his father's footsteps; he rejected the belief that illnesses were sent by the gods and that treatment must consist of appeasing them in the temple. Epilepsy, for example, was known as the 'sacred disease'; but Hippocrates was convinced that the cause lay within the brain. For him, good health came from inside, through a balance of the Alcmaeonic humors, and from outside through a healthy relationship between a person and his environment. It's a startlingly modern approach, and it's intriguing to notice that a comparable move away from superstition took place at around the same time on the other side of the world, in China. The *Huangdi Neijing* is a collection of texts written between the fifth and first centuries BCE which laid the foundations of modern Chinese medicine.

In contrast to Alcmaeon, Hippocrates is represented in the anatomist's library by more than sixty works on a wide range of specialities, known collectively as the Hippocratic Corpus. None of the volumes can be definitively attributed to Hippocrates himself; but most of them are contemporary with him, and most reflect the philosophy of the Hippocratic school. When one writes of a Hippocratic school, the reference is not only to a school of thought but also to an actual school which Hippocrates established on Kos. He was by all accounts a gifted teacher and it has been suggested that the

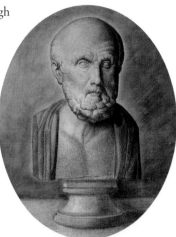

ABOVE

Hippocrates of Kos
(*c.*460–370 BCE)

The father of medicine, in whose name doctors traditionally took the Hippocratic Oath, swearing to do no intentional harm to their patients.

Hippocratic Corpus is all that remains of a much larger school library written by him and his pupils. Part of the historic value of the Hippocratic Corpus is that its authors reflect on their role and practice in the community, not only on their techniques.

Even in its diminished form it is an impressive reference collection. There are treatises on infection, disease and epidemics; on haemorrhoids and ulcers; on joint injuries, bone fractures and head trauma; and several volumes are devoted to gynaecology and urology. The various cavities and orifices of the body and the connections between them attracted considerable attention – there are books on enclosed channels (including sinews and blood vessels) and fistulae (abnormal connections between cavities). Although the existence of nerves had not yet been understood, Hippocrates is believed to have identified the vagus nerves which run from the brain down either side of the windpipe, which he referred to as 'two stout cords'.

Some works, including *On Anatomy*, are of a distinctly later date than the majority of the Hippocratic Corpus and may have been erroneously added by future compilers. Some have survived only in translation, in Arabic, Hebrew, Syriac or Latin. The earliest printed version of the Hippocratic Corpus, in Latin, was produced in 1525, giving it real shelf space in the anatomist's library. In modern languages, Dutch commentaries were published by the physician Franz Zacharias Ermerins in the mid-nineteenth century; and a French translation and commentary by Jacques Jouanna began in 1967. Although part of the Corpus had been available in English since 1597, the first full English translation was completed only in 2012.

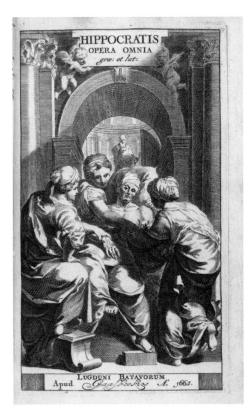

4 Pneuma, pulse and Praxagoras

Pneuma was an idea which gained some traction among followers of Hippocrates. It was an invisible life force which circulated the winds around the globe. Humans inhaled it by breathing; and in the body it propelled the humors to the major organs. It was a hard theory to refute; it was invisible, and when a patient stopped breathing they died, presumably from a critical lack of pneuma.

The school on Kos flourished and Hippocrates' students taught there or went out into the world to spread his teaching. Following Hippocrates' dictat that a knowledge of anatomy was essential for medical understanding, several Greek physicians made the art their focus of research. Diocles of Carystus (*c.*375–295 BCE) may have coined the term 'anatomy' and certainly wrote the first manual of animal anatomy. Neither it nor any of his other writing survives except as titles or quotations in the works of Galen and others. He was convinced that nerves were the communicators of sensation; and he is supposed to have invented the Spoon of Diocles, a surgical device for removing arrowheads from flesh and – on one occasion – the injured eye of Philip II of Macedon (father of Alexander the Great) from its socket.

Praxagoras (b. *c.*340 BCE) was born on Kos not long after the death of the school's founder and followed in his father's and grandfather's footsteps in becoming a physician. None of his writing survives; but again, we have Galen to thank for some knowledge of his work. Praxagoras drew a distinction between veins and arteries for the first time: veins, he deduced, carried blood, while arteries carried pneuma. It's no wonder that Galen questioned whether Praxagoras had actually conducted any dissections, although when Praxagoras examined the arteries of the deceased they were, admittedly, empty of blood. He thought that veins came from the liver and the arteries from the heart, and that arteries pulsed by themselves, not because of a heartbeat.

There are references throughout the Hippocratic Corpus to humors and pneuma; and Praxagoras subscribed to Alcmaeon's expanded list of the former. He thought, for example, that both epilepsy and paralysis were caused by an accumulation of congealed phlegm in the arteries, the result of a lack of heat. Both Diocles and Praxagoras disputed Alcmaeon's claim that the brain was the centre of reason; for them it was the heart which ruled. Nevertheless, Praxagoras's interest in the pulse promoted it as a useful diagnostic tool. His pupil Herophilos even wrote a treatise, *On Pulses*, which corrected Praxagoras's misapprehensions.

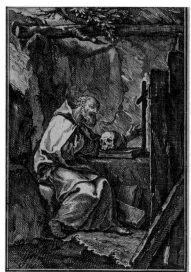

5 Herophilos, Erasistratus and Alexandria

Herophilos (*c.*335–280 BCE) was born on the coast of Turkey near Byzantium but moved to the exciting city of Alexandria in Egypt to pursue his education. Alexandria had been founded by Alexander the Great in Herophilos's lifetime (331 BCE) and was already emerging as a cosmopolitan centre of culture, a place where the wisdom of east and west, north and south met and became universal. It was, in the purest sense, a university of knowledge. Its famous library eventually held around 700,000 scrolls and it was there that the Hippocratic Corpus began to coalesce into a single body of work.

This critical mass of information attracted both teachers and pupils, and inspired an increased thirst for learning, especially in the field of medicine. It may have been for that reason that Alexandria was the only place in the civilised ancient world where the dissection of human cadavers was permitted: the desire for knowledge overrode the respect for custom. Herophilos took advantage of this permission to conduct the first extensive program of human anatomical investigation in history. He is today regarded as the founding father of anatomy.

Herophilos believed in an empirical approach to medicine, requiring the evidence of his own eyes. His corpses were those of criminals condemned to death; and writing in the time of Galen nearly 500 years later the early Christian author Tertullian claimed that Herophilos also conducted 600 vivisections of live prisoners. One assumes they were not invited to sign a consent form.

Herophilos wrote at least nine treatises, with subjects ranging from midwifery to the pulse, the latter perhaps a product of his work with living convicts. None of his works survive, but Galen's extensive admiring references to them in his own writings have preserved his memory and at least some of his ideas. Dissection was again taboo in Galen's lifetime and Galen relied heavily on Herophilos's luck in studying in the right place at the right time.

Herophilos's particular passions were the eye and the brain. He gave us the word 'retina' and believed, like Hippocrates, that the brain rather than the heart was the seat of thought processes. Herophilos was the first anatomist to identify motor and sensory nerves. He recognised the different functions of the cerebellum and the cerebrum, two different areas of the brain; and in the matter of veins and arteries he proved by dissection that both vessels carried only blood.

The advances in anatomy made by Herophilos were in large part responsible for Alexandria's reputation as a centre of medical excellence. Among his innovations was the measurement of pulse rate for diagnosis, using a water clock of his own invention. He could not, however, bring himself to refute the prevailing wisdom regarding humors and pneuma, which continued to have currency for the next 500 years. Blood, it was held, was a mixture of phlegm, black and yellow bile; and diagnosis could be made by drawing off and inspecting the blood of the patient.

Herophilos and a fellow physician Erasistratus of Keos (c.305–250 BCE) are often credited with founding the formal medical school in Alexandria, which emerged from the informal gatherings of teachers and students who congregated in the city. They were certainly its leading lights, and Erasistratus went on to establish a school of his own at Smyrna in Ionia which lasted for over 200 years.

Erasistratus is the subject of an apocryphal tale of diagnosis also told of Galen and

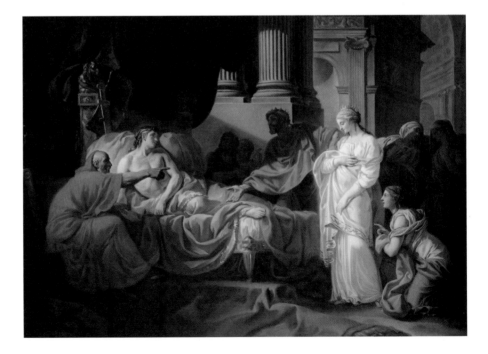

other physicians. He is said to have first revealed his aptitude for medicine when confronted with the mysterious ailment of Antiochus I Soter, son of King Seleucus I Nicator. Antiochus was wasting away with a disease which defied diagnosis, until Erasistratus noticed that his temperature rose, his pulse quickened and his colour deepened whenever the king's beautiful new wife Stratonice walked past. Antiochus was in love! Fearing to reveal the precise source of Antiochus's sickness, Erasistratus told the king that it was his own wife that the prince was besotted with. When the king tried to persuade Erasistratus to give Antiochus his wife, Erasistratus asked him if he would do the same were Stratonice the object of the lovestruck son's adoration. The king insisted that he would; and when Erasistratus revealed the truth, the king stuck to his word and gave Stratonice to his son along with a handful of provinces from his empire. The son eventually succeeded his father; and Erasistratus received a hundred talents for his diagnosis – one of the largest medical fees ever recorded. (Retellers of the story often omit the fact that Erasistratus would have been about ten years old at the time.)

Like Herophilos, Erasistratus was interested in the blood vessels, the nervous system and the brain. He observed a fourth ventricle of the brain where Herophilos had only seen three, and proposed that the greater surface area of the cerebral gyri in the human brain enabled man's greater intelligence compared to animals. He was thrillingly close to discovering the circulation of blood within the body: Galen quotes his observation that 'the vein arises from the part where the arteries, that are distributed to the whole body, have their origin, and penetrates to the sanguineous [right] ventricle; and the artery [pulmonary vein] arises from the part where the veins have their origin, and penetrates to the pneumatic [left] ventricle of the heart.'

After the deaths of Herophilos and Erasistratus the philosophy of the Alexandria medical school changed. Empiricism, a school of thought founded by one of Herophilos's students Philinus of Kos, became dominant. It held that dissection had no useful place in medicine and that perfectly good diagnosis and treatment could be made simply by non-invasive observation of the physical and mental state of a patient. Human dissection fell out of favour. A war with Syria in the third and second centuries BCE drained the city's resources and brought intellectuals under suspicion. Instead of practical research and experiment, physicians retreated into literary scholarship, studying only the works of their predecessors and abandoning potentially unpopular innovation. Alexandria lost much of its status as a global centre of excellence and anatomy made no real advances until Claudius Galenus turned his inquiring mind to the subject in the second century CE.

6 Galen

Galen (129–216 CE) was born in Pergamon, the modern-day town of Bergama in Turkey. The location is significant because it was the site of an asclepeion, a temple dedicated to Asclepius, the Greek god of healing. It was also an intellectual and cultural centre whose library of manuscripts was rivalled only by that of Alexandria. Leading figures travelled to Pergamon for learning or cures.

Words, knowledge and medicine were Galen's childhood playground. His father raised him to be a politician and as a boy Galen was exposed to the various schools of philosophical thought of the day. When he was sixteen, however, Asclepius appeared in a

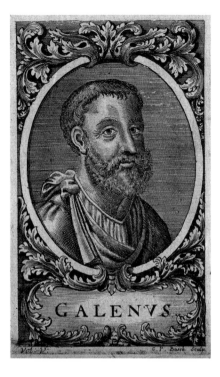

dream to his father, ordering him to educate his son in the healing arts. Galen therefore attended the asclepeion in Pergamon where, working as a junior therapy attendant, he was taught medicine for four years. One of his tutors was the empiric pharmacist Aescrion, whose cure for the bite of a mad dog Galen later recalled admiringly. It required crayfish to be caught during a particular phase of the sun and moon, and to be baked alive, then ground into a powder – presumably for the high levels of calcium and phosphates in their exoskeletons.

Having completed his training in Pergamon, Galen took to the road travelling around the Mediterranean as a journeyman physician. He visited medical schools and centres at Smyrna (perhaps the one established by Erasistratus), on the islands of Cyprus and Crete, the Greek mainland and in southern Turkey, before finally migrating to Alexandria. There he soaked up all that the great library could offer of the works of Alcmaeon, Hippocrates, Herophilos and others.

He returned to Pergamon at the age of twenty-eight to take up a post as physician to the gladiators of the rich and prominent High Priest of Asia. In a role equivalent to team doctor his job was to patch up the injuries with which so many of the gladiators came off the field of combat. Galen later claimed that his employer set a tough test for applicants for the position. He killed an ape, removed all its vital organs, then invited the job hopefuls to reassemble the unfortunate creature like a jigsaw without a picture.

Deprived of the legal opportunity to dissect human cadavers, Galen had plenty of occasion to see the insides of his charges through open wounds, which he described as 'windows into the body'. He served in the post for four years, during which only five gladiators died of their injuries, compared to sixty under the previous jobholder. With this experience, and the boost to his confidence it must have given him, Galen felt bold enough to move to the centre of the western world, Rome. There he built a solid reputation not only as a physician but as a showman. He regularly staged public dissections of animals including fish, snakes, ostriches and – on at least one occasion – an elephant, which he bought from the city's Circus Maximus.

His evident medical talent was not universally welcomed in Rome. Established physicians felt threatened by this new arrival, and he was warned that on a previous occasion they had poisoned a rival and his entourage. Galen therefore left Rome for a while but was summoned back to the city in 169 CE by the emperor himself, Marcus Aurelius. Roman troops returning from a war in the north had brought smallpox back with them and an epidemic was raging, sometimes known to historians as Galen's Plague. Galen was to join the imperial court as its physician, accompanying Marcus Aurelius and his co-emperor Lucius Verus when they returned to the battlefront. Galen was reluctant to go, and eventually a message reached Marcus Aurelius that the god Asclepius – once again overseeing Galen's career – was opposed to the idea. It was for the best: Lucius Verus died of the disease later that year and the epidemic persisted for many years, claiming Marcus Aurelius, too, in 180 CE.

Instead, Galen was ordered to remain in Rome to attend Marcus Aurelius's son and heir Commodus. He took advantage of the ample free time which his duties must have afforded him to write many of his medical works during this period. He continued to serve Commodus when he became emperor but was unable to save him from a successful assassination attempt – a gladiatorial wrestler drowned Commodus in the bath. After a turbulent year of civil war and rival claims to the imperial laurels, Galen displayed impressive political survival skills by becoming physician to the eventual victor and new emperor Septimius Severus and his son Caracalla. He probably retired to Sicily where his remains may still be buried – his tomb in Palermo was still standing in the tenth century.

Galen was undoubtedly a gifted physician and surgeon, celebrated in his own lifetime. His success was built on his willingness to learn both from the writing of others and from his own experiments. In return he left behind an enormous legacy of written works on a wide range of medical and philosophical topics. By some estimates this one man was responsible for almost half of the entire surviving body of ancient Greek texts. Unlike Hippocrates' canon, the Galenic corpus was entirely written by Galen. Even during his own life he was subject to forgeries, and in response he wrote *De libris propriis* (*On My Own Books*) which lists his authentic works with a synopsis and context for each one, providing many autobiographical details. It serves as a catalogue not only of his own books but as a reference to the many other anatomists whom he credited or criticised.

Several of Galen's books are on anatomical matters. *De anatomicis administrationibus* (On Anatomical Procedures) and *De usu partium corporis humani* (Of the Functions of the Different Parts of the Human Body) are his best-known general works in the field. Like earlier anatomists he was interested in the reproductive system, observed through treatises *De semine* (On Semen), *De foetuum formatione* (On Foetal Formation) and *De uteri dissectione* (On the Dissection of the Uterus) – the latter unfortunately based on his examination of canine anatomy which differs from the human form in this and other respects.

Galen also turned his attention to the circulatory system. In his *An in arteriis natura sanguis contineatur (Is Blood Naturally Contained in the Arteries?)* he concluded with a resounding yes, not oxygen – the prevailing doctrine. He was the first anatomist to comment on the difference between venous (dark red) and arterial (bright red) blood and concluded that there were two distinct circulation systems in the body. He proposed the veins carried blood which originated in the kidneys (as Hippocrates had thought) and the arteries brought different blood from and to the heart. The theory was only refuted more than a thousand years later. In addition, he correctly proposed a third system, that of nerves responsible for sensation and thought centred on the brain.

Some of his most important and accurate work was done on the spine. Through experiments with live pigs he established the effect of cutting the spinal cord in different places. They gave him a good working knowledge of the human spine and of the impact of nerve damage on muscles, which he was the first to differentiate as agonists (that is, muscles which make movement) and antagonists (those which inhibit it).

Galen was unable to abandon the prevalent theories of humors and pneuma, perhaps for fear of appearing too revolutionary. Instead he distinguished between psychic pneuma, running through the nervous system, and vital pneuma which coursed through the arteries of the heart. It's easy to scoff at the ideas of early anatomists but they were pioneers in the field. Galen, through his scientific method of informed experiment, came to a greater understanding of anatomy than anyone before him; and, as it turned out, than any who came after him over the following millennium.

7 Decline and Fall of the Western Empire

On My Own Books is a good starting place for an overview of Galen's contributions to anatomy. As well as its autobiographical elements, it contains fascinating observations on the medical events and practices of the day, and references to the philosophies and anatomical assumptions of times before Galen's. Galen recorded all that historical information, preserving the ideas and lost works of the past; and yet original versions of Galen's own work are as absent from the anatomist's library as those to which he refers.

Two disastrous fires and a dramatic shift in the world order are responsible for the loss of as much as two-thirds of Galen's work. The first fire happened in his lifetime and while he was living nearby. Rome's Temple of Peace was built (like so many monuments to peace) in the aftermath, and with the profits, of a war – in this case, Rome's sack of Jerusalem in 70 CE by the emperor Vespasian. In *On My Own Books* Galen describes the fire which engulfed it in 192. It was rebuilt by his patron Septimius Severus a decade later, but several of Galen's works were destroyed in the event.

The same temple was finally left to ruin after it sustained serious damage during the Sack of Rome by the Visigoths of northern Europe in 410. It had probably been closed down thirty years earlier when the Edict of Thessalonica adopted Christianity as the official religion of the Roman Empire. Pagan worshippers became the objects of

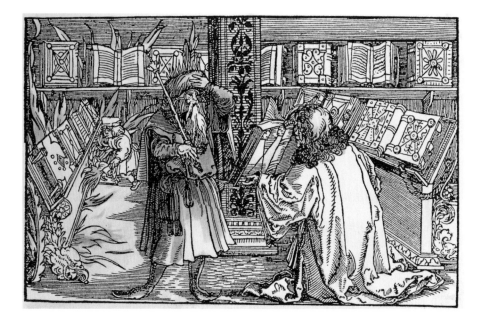

persecution just as the early Christians had once been. By then the Roman Empire had been divided administratively into east and west, with imperial courts in both Rome and Constantinople.

While the Eastern Empire flourished, and as the Holy Roman Empire persisted until the sixteenth century, the Western Empire was in terminal decline. Emperor Theodosius (who introduced the Edict of Thessalonica) fought and won a punishing series of wars against the Goths but these and internal factions left the forces of Roman law and order greatly depleted in western Europe. In the absence of any central authority the Western Empire was broken up into small kingdoms by local warlords.

One of the early victims of the decline of the Roman Empire was the great Library at Alexandria, where Galen and his predecessors studied. Alexandria's original importance to Rome as a centre of learning and source of grain decreased as other libraries were established around the Mediterranean and other parts of the empire were opened up to farming. Where once scholars had been paid to teach and research, underfunding now reduced the institution to little more than a couple of warehouses for hundreds of thousands of dusty scrolls.

There was no single catastrophic conflagration that finally destroyed the Library at Alexandria. It survived Julius Caesar, who accidentally set fire to part of it in 48 BCE. It was rebuilt after that and, as it outgrew its original building, a temple, the Serapeum, was co-opted as a second home for some of the Library's collection. Gradually, however, administrative neglect and a decline in status took their toll. The Serapeum survived the probable destruction of the main library building in around 275 CE during a battle for control of the city between Roman and Palmyrian forces. But, as a pagan temple, it could not withstand the Christianisation of the Roman Empire which decreed, in 391, that it be demolished and its contents destroyed. Any of the Library's surviving Galenic texts were finally lost at that time.

8 Move to the East

In the west, these major events accompanied the descent into the so-called Dark Ages. Without the stability of Roman civilisation, the arts and sciences fell into decline and the centre of intellectual activity moved eastwards to Constantinople. Galen's importance remained undiminished and in the Eastern Empire it became an influence on Islamic thought. Soon after his death, and in the centuries which followed it, many of his surviving works were translated into Arabic, Farsi and Syriac; and while in the western world science retreated into the philosophical study of ancient texts, the flame of anatomical enquiry was kept burning in the Middle East.

Of particular importance in this respect is Hunayn ibn Ishāq (809–873), an enthusiastic translator who travelled widely in the Middle East looking for old works. As a physician he was aware of Galen's reputation and translated over a hundred of his works into Arabic including several of anatomical interest – *De ossibus* (*On Bones for Beginners*), *De anatomicis administrationibus* (*On Anatomical Procedures*), and treatises on the voice, the chest and lungs, the eye and other parts. Ishāq subsequently published his own series, *Ten Treatises of the Eye*, which includes the first ever anatomical diagram of that organ.

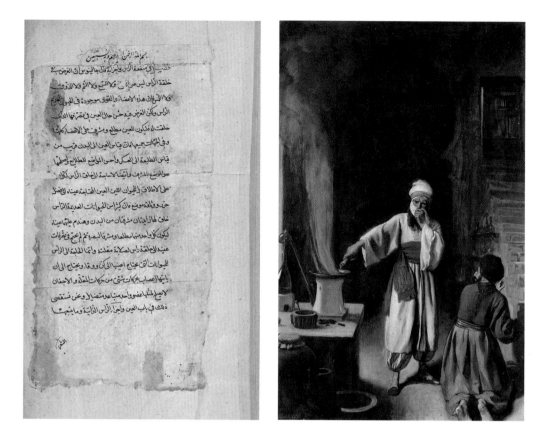

9 Rhazes

Coming a few decades after Ishāq and certainly benefiting from the availability of his translations, Abū Bakr Muhammad bin Zakariyā al-Rāzī (known by his latinised name Rhazes) is an under-celebrated hero of medical history. He was a follower of Hippocrates and Galen, committed to practical experimental research, who made discoveries of his own. Rhazes (*c*.864–935) lived in the region of modern-day Tehran. He was a polymath of considerable intellect who wrote over 200 texts on subjects from grammar to astronomy. Works on alchemy and philosophy sit alongside many on medical and anatomical matters which, when translated into Latin, had a considerable influence on western thinking as Europe began to emerge from its Dark Age slumber.

As chief physician of Baghdad Rhazes was a noted teacher and a committed healer of all parts of the community. Among his many books was *Man la yahduruhu al-tabib* (*For One Who Has No Physician to Attend Him*), probably the world's first household medical handbook, aimed at those who through poverty or remoteness could not consult a doctor in person. He was a fierce critic of charlatans and snake-oil salesmen who preyed on the poor. Another book, *Al-Hawi* (*The Virtuous Life*), was a comprehensive teaching textbook in twenty-three volumes, assembled by his students from his notes after his death.

His contributions to medicine are extensive. He produced the first treatise dealing specifically with ailments of children, for which he is regarded as the father of paediatrics. He wrote authoritatively on smallpox and, like Ishāq, was fascinated by the human eye – he was the first to notice the reaction of the pupil to bright light. Cruelly, Rhazes struggled with failing eyesight himself; it is said that he refused to be operated on for the condition because his doctors could not answer his testing questions about ophthalmic anatomy. Through Rhazes, Galen's ideas travelled even further east; he read Galen aloud to a Chinese student of his, who copied them down verbatim in Chinese. And when Rhazes' own works were translated into Latin and introduced to medieval Europe, one edition of *The Virtuous Life* was edited and annotated by Andreas Vesalius, the father of modern anatomy.

Rhazes regarded one of his most important works as a heretical and regrettable necessity. He prefaced *Al-Shukūk ʿalā Jalīnūs* (*Doubts About Galen*) with high praise for the man 'whose status is so awesome, whose rank is so majestic, whose legacy is so universal, and whose memory is revered so eternally.' But he continued, 'the discipline of medicine and philosophy does not allow us to submit blindly to prominent leaders or to comply with them, or to avoid thoroughly investigating [their views], and no philosopher would want his readers and students to do that. Galen himself said that in his book *On the Usefulness of the Parts of the Body*.'

Not all Rhazes' criticism was anatomical. He objected, naturally enough, to Galen's assertion that Greek was the best language; and he felt that Galen had less experience of the diseases which he observed than Rhazes did. Coming from a different tradition, Rhazes was highly critical of Galen's adherence to the humors. He pointed out that simply drinking a hot or cold drink was enough to upset the supposed balance of humors and suggested that the body was reacting to temperature rather than any imagined bile or phlegm. He also disputed Aristotle's earth, air, fire and water theory, the roots of Galen's humors; as an alchemist he found that those four elements alone could not explain many of the qualities of matter such as sulphurousness or salinity.

He was in a sense proposing the existence of the chemical elements as we understand them today, something that wasn't accepted until the late seventeenth century when Robert Boyle again challenged Aristotle's view. In Rhazes' time he was considered an arrogant fool for daring to question Galen; today there is some justification in regarding him as the greatest physician of the medieval era.

10 Avicenna

The first great medical book of the second millennium CE was written by Rhazes' countryman Ibn Sīnā, latinised as Avicenna (980–1037). His five-volume *Al-Qanun fi't-Tibb* (*Canon of Medicine*), completed in 1025, pulled together medical traditions from Greece, Rome, Asia and China and remained a standard medical reference work in both Europe and the Islamic world well into the eighteenth century.

The Canon of Medicine owes much to Galen, including its adherence to the humors, which he believed formed, in different combinations, the different parts of the anatomy. Bone, for example, had a greater proportion of black bile, while the brain was dominated by phlegm. He expanded on the concept by allowing each humor a degree of warmth or

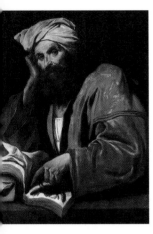

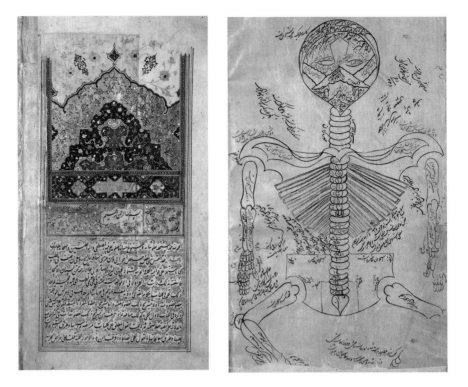

coolness, softness or hardness and dryness or wetness. Furthermore, he proposed four
types of spirit which connected the impure body to the pure soul: brutal spirit, located in
the heart and the source of all the others; sensual, in the brain; natural, in the liver; and
procreative, found in the testes and ovaries. In the heart-versus-brain debate Avicenna
concurred with Aristotle that the heart was the seat of reason.

Book Three of the *Canon* is a comprehensive anatomy of the human body from top
to toe. It is more concerned with how disease affects the various parts rather than directly
with the physiology of the parts themselves. It shows a quite modern understanding of
many conditions including cataracts of the eye, strokes and narrowing of the arteries.
Avicenna is advanced in his grasp of the nervous system and his treatment of a broad
range of neurological disorders from nervous tics to epilepsy, and sciatica to meningitis.

11 Ibn al-Nafis

Avicenna was constrained, like many of his predecessors, by moral objections to human
dissection, and he followed Galen in assuming that apes were a close substitute. He and
Rhazes were part of an Islamic Golden Age of learning centred on Baghdad, the largest
city in the world at the time. The place was home to the House of Wisdom, a library
established by the caliph Harun al-Rashid (763–809) who gave orders that it be filled
with the translated knowledge of the world. It was in every sense a new Alexandria and it
lasted for nearly 500 years until Baghdad was sacked by the Mongols in 1258. It is said

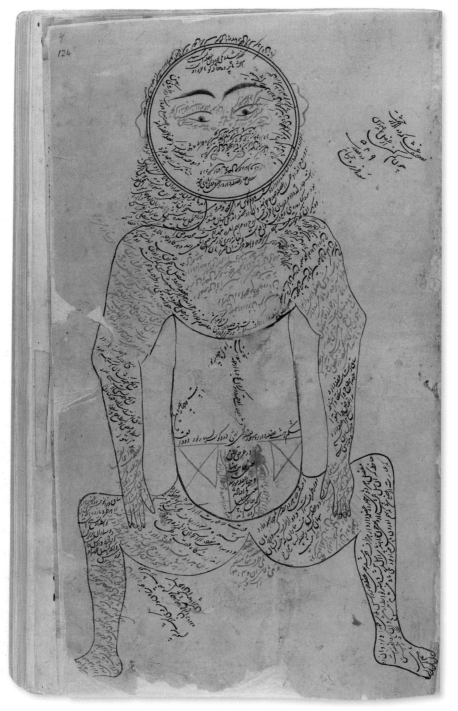

LEFT

The Canon of Medicine

Avicenna's drawing of the
muscular system of the
human body.

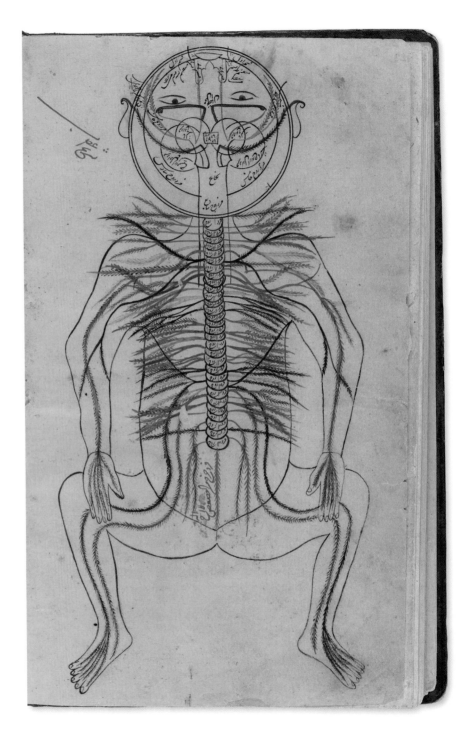

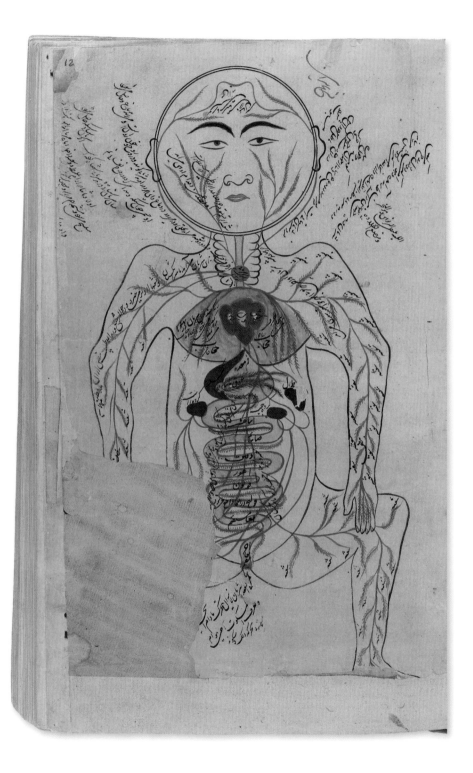

LEFT

The Canon of Medicine

Avicenna's illustration of the arteries and viscera of the human body.

that the River Tigris ran red with blood and black with the ink of books from the House of Wisdom that were thrown into it.

The Golden Age's anatomical last hurrah was in the works of Ibn al-Nafis (1213–88). The celebrated physician spent most of his life in Egypt and thereby avoided first-hand experience of the fall of Baghdad, when the city was razed and its citizens massacred. Ibn al-Nafis had the advantage over Rhazes and Avicenna of being able to experiment on human cadavers, through which he made the significant discovery of pulmonary circulation, far in advance of similar 'discoveries' in the west. At the time of his death, he had only completed eighty of a projected 300 volumes of his masterwork *Al-Shamil fi al-Tibb* (*The Comprehensive Book on Medicine*), fragments of which survive in libraries around the world, including two complete volumes still in Egypt.

Of special interest to anatomists are his commentaries on Hippocrates' *On the Nature of Man* and on Avicenna's various works on anatomy. Ibn al-Nafis echoes Hippocrates' tenet that a good knowledge of anatomy was vital for any physician, something he demonstrates by subsequently setting out his own excellent grasp of the subject. In addition to his discovery of pulmonary circulation, he also made breakthroughs in the understanding of the coronary and capillary circulation systems. More than anyone else during the Islamic Golden Age, Ibn al-Nafis moved the study of anatomy beyond the philosophical limitations of its earlier Greco-Roman orthodoxy.

Discovery of the 'small circulation' by Ibn al Nafis (1213–88)

Ibn al-Nafis suggested in the thirteenth-century that blood in the right ventricle passes through the lungs and is aerated there before entering the left ventricle.

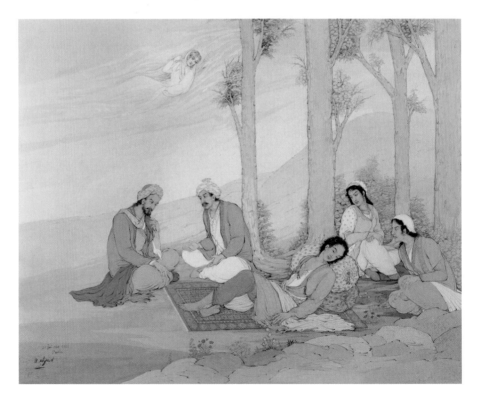

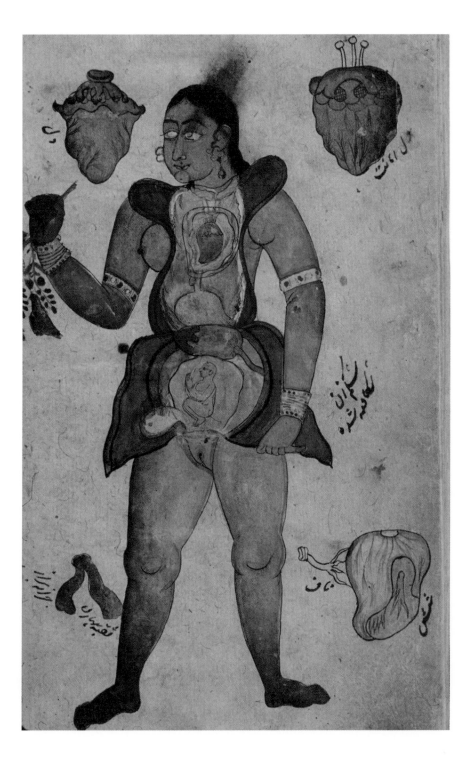

Akbar's Medicine

Female anatomy, from an
eighteenth-century Indian
copy of a Persian commentary
by Mohammed Akbar on an
earlier commentary by Burhan-
ud-din Kermani on an even
earlier work, Najib ad-Din
Samarqandi's thirteenth-
century *Book of Causes
and Symptoms*.

RIGHT

Akbar's Medicine

Male anatomy, from a
commentary on Najib ad-Din
Samarqandi's thirteenth-
century *Book of Causes and
Symptoms*, shows the lasting
impact of the Golden Age of
Islamic medicine.

OPPOSITE

Akbar's Medicine

Left: Details of the male and
female reproductive systems,
derived from *The Book of
Causes and Symptoms*. Above
right: Rear view of a male
skeleton. In addition to his
commentaries, Mohammed
Akbar (sometimes known as
Muqim Arzani) wrote many
original treatises on diseases of
pregnancy and infancy, and on
medicinal compounds. Below
right: The viscera, including
the liver and gall bladder
(upper left), and the stomach
and intestines (centre).

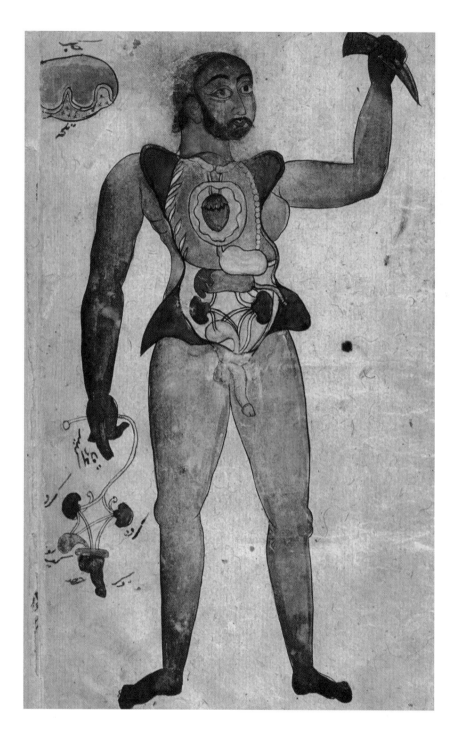

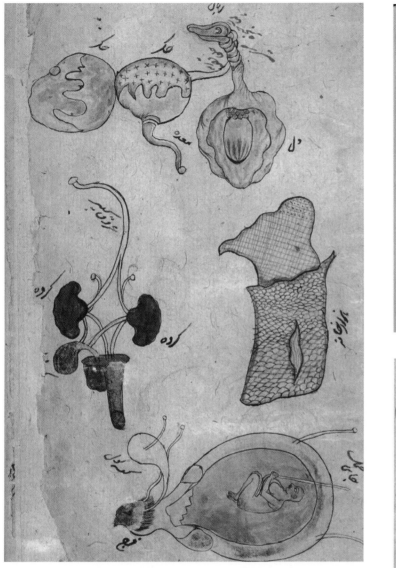

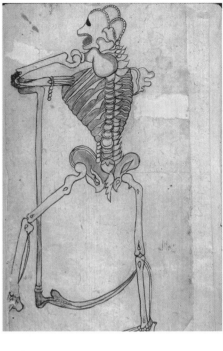

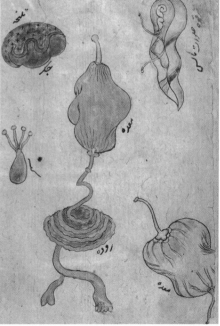

Front view of a male skeleton. Little is known of Najib ad-Din Samarqandi, on whose work Akbar's is based. He died in 1222 during the Mongol sacking of Herat, an Afghani centre of learning.

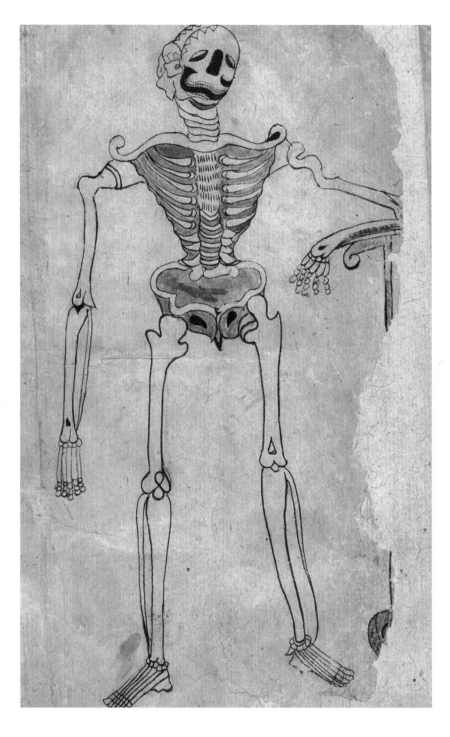

12 Return to Western Europe

The twelfth and thirteenth centuries saw the start of an intellectual revival in western Europe. Universities were founded, first at Bologna in Italy (in 1088, with a charter granted in 1158) and Paris in France (1150) and by 1300 at Oxford and Cambridge in England and many cities throughout France, Italy and Spain. The word 'university' was coined for the Bologna institution.

The scarcity of study material in the form of Greek and Roman literature drove the universities to look beyond Europe, prompting a wave of translations of Islamic works, and of Greek and Roman works earlier translated into Arabic back into Latin. Since many of the original works had by now been forgotten or lost, these new translations of old ideas formed the core of a new scientific lexicon.

Some of the Arabic originals made their way to western Europe by way of the Islamic conquests of Spain and Sicily. Toledo in central Spain, for example, had become a centre of learning under Muslim occupation and remained a multicultural treasure trove of manuscripts after Alfonso VI of León and Castile recaptured the city for Christianity in 1085. It was to Toledo that one Gerard of Cremona made a linguistic pilgrimage in the mid-twelfth century, hoping to learn Arabic so that he could read a copy of Ptolemy's *Almagest* kept in the city.

The *Almagest*, a primary scientific text on mathematics and astronomy, had a formidable reputation among scholars, although most had not read it because it had not yet been translated into Latin. Gerard, thus introduced to the treasures of Toledo's libraries in search of this one text, spent the remainder of his life in the city enthusiastically translating all the scientific works that he could lay his eyes on. He brought Rhazes' work to the attention of the Christian world; and he (or another translator with the same name working a century later) translated Avicenna's *Canon of Medicine*.

Toledo attracted a veritable posse of translators, drawn not only by the presence of the source material but by the proximity of the Islamic, Jewish and Christian communities within the city. Christian translators often worked alongside native Arabic or Hebrew speakers. They congregated in Toledo Cathedral and worked almost feverishly to bring knowledge to a Latin-speaking readership. The Toledo School of Translators effected a dissemination of scientific, philosophical and religious thought on a scale which, relatively speaking, would not be seen again until the invention of the internet. Gerard alone translated eighty-seven books. Perhaps because of the dates in which he was working, after the establishment of the Toledo School and at the end of the Golden Age, Ibn al-Nafis escaped the attention of translators until the fourteenth century and remained largely overlooked until his work on pulmonary circulation was rediscovered in the early twentieth century.

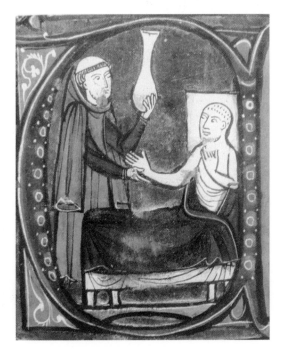

BELOW

Examining urine

Attributed to Aldobrandino of Siena (d. *c.*1299) whose book *Le Régime du Corps* (*The Regulation of the Body*) was published in 1256. The colour, substance, contents and quantity of a patient's urine were considered useful diagnostic aids.

13 Frederick II

Translation was not confined to Toledo. Frederick II of Sicily (1194–1250), a remarkable man of broad intellectual interests, spoke six languages himself, including Latin, Greek and Arabic; and he ordered translators to scour the known world for texts. By promoting the literary use of the Sicilian language in his royal court in Palermo he laid the foundations of modern Italian. Among the many sciences in which he took an interest, anatomy seems particularly to have caught his imagination. Contemporary records describe a number of cruel experiments with prisoners. In one case he sealed a man in a barrel in the hope of seeing the prisoner's soul escape through the bung hole at the moment of death. In another he fed two prisoners an identical meal and sent one to bed and the other one hunting; he then disembowelled both to compare the effects of sloth and activity on their digestive systems.

In 1224 Frederick founded the University of Sicily, having by then added the thrones of Italy, Germany and the Holy Roman Empire to his name; and in 1231, now also King of Jerusalem, he ordained that anatomy be a compulsory part of the curriculum for every medical student and so, for that purpose, a human body should be dissected for their benefit every five years.

BELOW

**Frederick II of Sicily
(1194–1250)**

In a painting by Giacomo Conti (1813–88), philosopher Michael Scotus of the Toledo School presents his translation of the works of Aristotle to the king in the Royal Palace at Palermo.

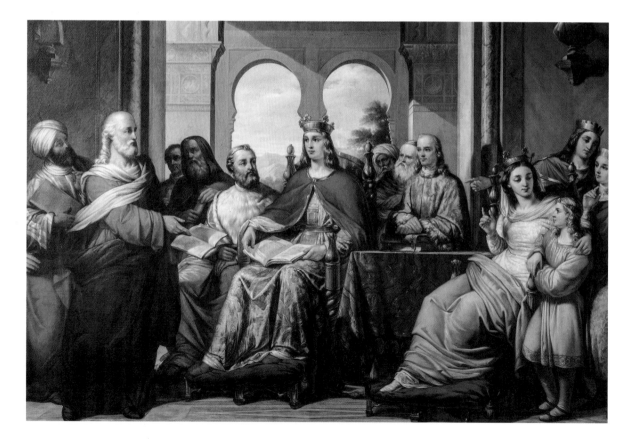

It's difficult to overstate the impact of this decree on the science of anatomy, which had been hampered by the need to guess at human physiology based on the dissection of dogs, pigs and monkeys for thousands of years. By the time of his death in 1250, Frederick II was already being hailed as the Wonder of the Age for his spirit of inquiry; and Friedrich Nietzsche in the nineteenth century described him as the first European, for the efficient, centralised bureaucracy of his government of Sicily. History does not record whether or not, on his entombment in a porphyry sarcophagus in Palermo Cathedral, his soul was seen to escape, but rumours persisted for years that he was not dead, only sleeping.

Although resistance to the idea of human dissection persisted it was, thanks to Frederick II, legalised in much of Europe over the next 130 years. The earliest examples on record were autopsies conducted to determine the cause of death of individuals. The first known human dissection of the modern age took place in Cremona in 1286. The universities of Paris and Bologna emerged as the leading centres of anatomical study; and it was at the latter, in January 1315, that an event took place which marked the science's modern beginnings.

Mondino de Luzzi (1270–1326), a former student of the University of Bologna and now a lecturer in surgery, performed – in a theatrical sense, before an audience – the first public dissection of a human cadaver, probably a female one. The following year he wrote a manual for the practice, *Anathomia corporis humani* (*The Anatomy of the Human Body*). Although it was not published until 1478, after the invention of movable type, it remained in print for a hundred years thereafter and is sometimes credited as the first modern anatomy book.

It was, in truth, not all that modern; much of its thinking, despite his practical experience, still reflected for the most part the ideas of Galen and Avicenna. But it can claim to be the first book whose subject was completely and solely the science of anatomy. So this book, with its knowledge of the past and the very practical approach of its present, is the first modern volume in the anatomist's library.

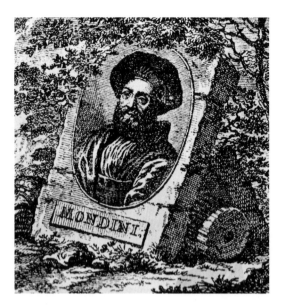

ABOVE

Mondino de Luzzi (1270–1326)

Revered as the physician who reintroduced the study of anatomy to Europe, Mondino is said to have conducted the first public dissection of modern times.

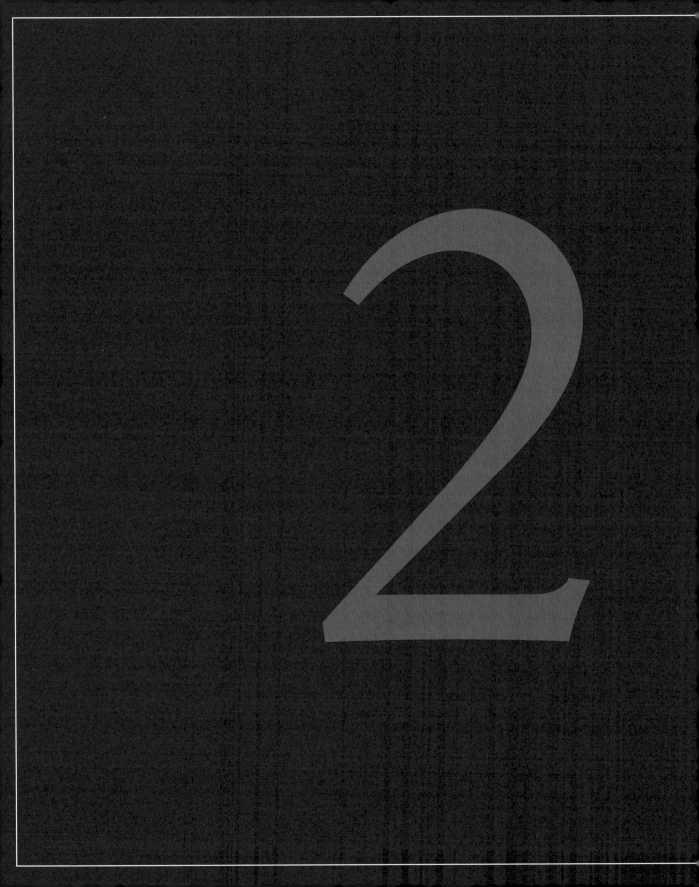

MEDIEVAL
ANATOMY

1301–1500

One of the first anatomy books to be printed, rather than transcribed by hand, ran to at least forty editions and was required reading in anatomy schools for 300 years after its author's death. It contains no dogma, no philosophy, no broader medical principles. It simply explains anatomy for anatomists.

1 Mondino de Luzzi

Anathomia corporis humani (*The Anatomy of the Human Body*) was written Mondino de Luzzi (1270–1326) in 1316 and published in 1475. The great advantage of the advent of the printing press, beside the overall ease of reproduction, was the facility to include illustrations – not the colourful, artful illuminations of monastic texts, but images which supported and reinforced the words. Although early editions of *Anathomia* only carried his text, within fifteen years images had been added. Previously pictures had to be laboriously copied by hand by scribes who did not necessarily understand what they were copying. The illustrations of Mondino's text amplify not only the anatomy of the body but his process of dissection. He ranked three areas of the body from least to most noble – the abdomen contained lowly 'natural members' such as the stomach and liver; the thorax housed the 'spiritual members' including the heart and lungs; and the skull contained the superior 'animal members' like the eyes and ears and the brain. His dissections, and his book, began in the nether regions with a vertical incision across the stomach and a horizontal one just above the navel – and an illustration shows very graphically how this should look with the skin peeled back to reveal its contents.

The book proceeds to deal with the organs in the order in which they are encountered – intestines first, then stomach, and so on. His descriptions are in some cases remarkably accurate – of the vena cava, for example, which brings deoxygenated blood back to the heart in circulation, and of the pulmonary artery and vein. But he adheres to an Aristotelian belief that the heart had three chambers – the right and left ventricles and a middle chamber concealed within the septum (the wall between the ventricles). The right ventricle, he insisted, drew blood produced in the liver; the left was filled with a smoky vapour from the lungs. A vital spirit, equivalent to the pneuma, was (he asserted) produced in the middle chamber. He makes no mention of the right and left atria, through which the blood enters and leaves the heart.

Even worse is his view of the uterus. It echoed a theory which had already been challenged in Bologna before his time. It was believed in the early Middle Ages that the uterus had seven chambers or cells in which foetuses could develop; three on the right produced male children, three on the left females and one in the middle was reserved for the gestation of hermaphrodites. Here, surely, was a misconception which could have been disproved easily by dissection? Mondino's repetition of the error undermines his claim to have dissected two women's bodies. Although some historians claim that Mondino conducted his own dissections, such

Anathomia corporis humani (1475)

Below: The title page from Mondino's posthumously published textbook shows the master anatomist instructing an inattentive *sector*. Opposite: The anatomy of a pregnant woman, from Mondino's classic book.

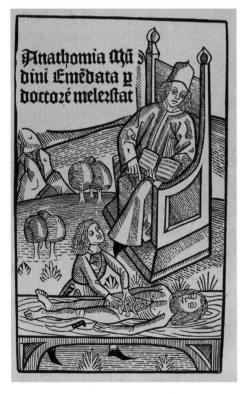

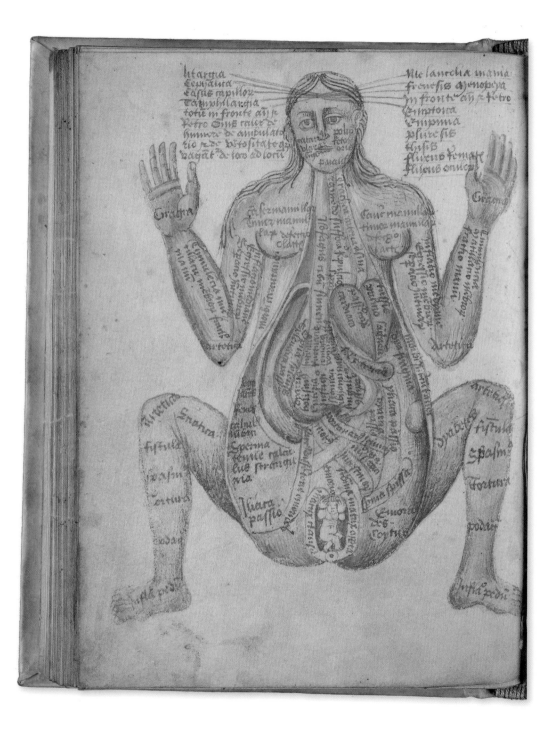

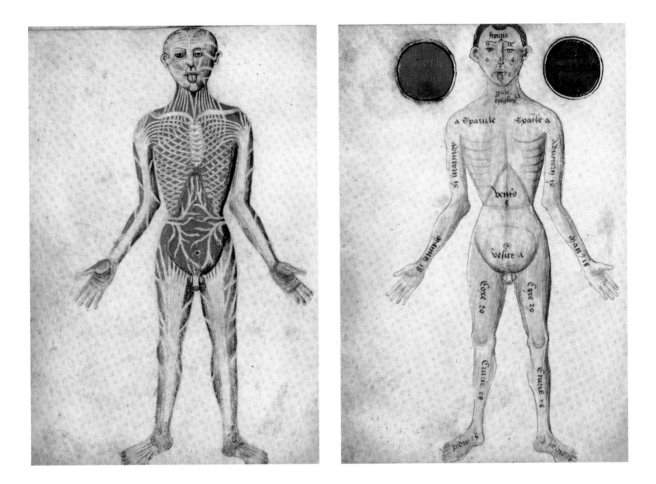

public demonstrations were not usually performed by the anatomist himself. Rather, he would narrate proceedings from a podium, often merely reading aloud the stages of the process from a book, as if describing the scenes of a play to confused members of its audience. Three people were involved in the performance: the *lector* (reader, in Latin) described the anatomy from his book and lofty position; the *sector* (cutter) made the actual incisions and excisions in the body; and an *ostensor* (indicator) used a pointed stick, like a teacher at a blackboard, to draw the audience's attention to the parts which the *sector* had revealed and which the *lector* was currently talking about. It's a setting which recalls a priest in his pulpit, delivering a sermon: the word of the *lector*, like the bible of a *rector*, is supreme. The truth, for the audience, is what the *lector* tells them, not the evidence of their or the *sector's* eyes. Indeed, in the image of a public dissection from a 1493 edition of *Anathomia*, the public don't seem to be looking at the corpse at all.

Despite its inaccuracies, Mondino's *Anathomia corporis humani* is a landmark publication. It treats anatomy as a science, not an illustration of philosophy. Although it repeated some Hippocratic and Galenic fallacies, it corrected some others and can be regarded as the first modern anatomy book, the founding volume of any modern anatomist's library.

2 Guido da Vigevano

Although illustrations accompanied later editions of *Anathomia*, it was a student of Mondino, Guido da Vigevano (1280–1349), who pioneered their use in anatomy. Guido is a fascinating character, a polymath carved – admittedly rather crudely – from the same stone as Leonardo da Vinci. He was a physician, an inventor, a diplomat, an Italian who wrote books about war machinery and anatomy dedicated to Philippe VI of France. After his studies in Bologna he practiced medicine in his native Pavia, in Lombardy, before being appointed court physician to the Holy Roman Emperor, Henry VII.

Medieval northern Italy was the battleground of the Guelphs and Ghibellines, two factions which supported, respectively, the authorities of the Pope and the Holy Roman Emperor. Henry VII's reign was defined by his political and military conflict with Robert of Naples, a captain in the Guelph League. Pope Clement V backed Robert; and when Henry died during a siege of the Guelph city of Siena in 1313, Clement issued a papal interdict against Ghibelline towns such as Pavia. Interdicts withdrew the spiritual benefits of the Catholic church from individuals and populations, denying them the comforts of, for example, absolution from sins and burial in consecrated ground. An interdict could also have more temporal consequences in damaging trade and withholding political protection.

Guido da Vigevano's membership of Henry's inner court made him something of a target and he fled to France, where his credentials gained him employment as personal physician to Jeanne of Burgundy, and subsequently to her husband, King Philippe VI of

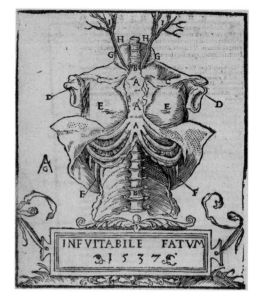

Anathomia corporis humani (1475)

Opposite: The blood vessels (left) and the muscles (right) of the male anatomy, from Mondino's book. The circles represent the four ventricles of the brain which were thought to exist. Above: A dissected male torso, in an illustration that shows not only the anatomy but Mondino's process of dissection.

RIGHT

Texaurus regis Francie (1335)

Guido de Vigevano's proposal
for a flotation device to enable
knights on horseback to
cross rivers.

OPPOSITE

*Anathomia Philippi
Septimi* (1345)

The first incision of a
dissection, from Guido de
Vigevano's work dedicated
to Philip VI of France.

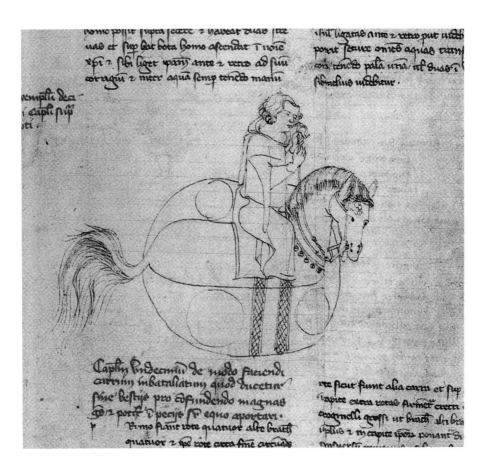

France. Philippe's claim to the French throne rested on a change to French law which excluded his more entitled rival, Edward III of England, on the grounds that Edward was descended from a female line. Philippe and Edward nevertheless planned to conduct a crusade together and, in support of it, Guido wrote his *Texaurus regis Francie* (*A Thesaurus for the King of France*) in 1335. It was a catalogue of proposals for the machinery of siege warfare, including armoured vehicles, temporary bridges, wind-powered carts and towers for assaulting city walls. Tensions between Edward and Philippe arose, however, and the crusade never took place. Instead, they fought the Hundred Years War against each other.

Guido's other two books may have been of more practical use to Philippe. He complied a medical handbook, *Regimen sanitatis* (*Health Manual*), to accompany the king on his crusade. It paid particular attention to the threats to health of the eastern Mediterranean climate, and to the risks which the leader of a crusade might face – there is a special section on the antidotes to poisons used by assassins. Guido had tried at least one of them on himself; having noticed that caterpillars fed on deadly wolfsbane with impunity, Guido ate some roots of the plant and then ingested a purée of the larvae. He survived, to write not only the *Regimen sanitatis* but his own contribution to the

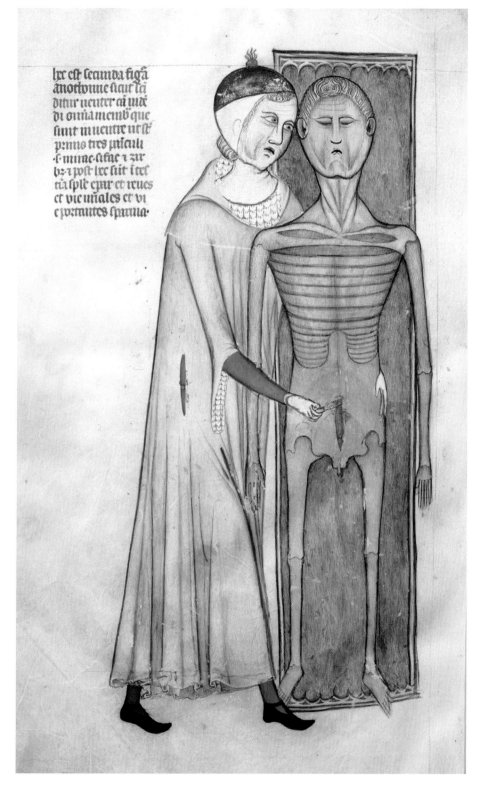

Anathomia Philippi
Septimi (1345)

An anatomist opens the skull
of a corpse with a hammer
and scalpel, a process known
as trephination.

OPPOSITE

Anathomia Philippi
Septimi (1345)

Above left: Female anatomy
showing the Galenic belief that
the uterus had seven chambers
– three for male babies, three
for female babies and one for
hermaphrodites. Above right:
The thoracic and abdominal
viscera of the male anatomy.
Below left: The digestive
system of the male anatomy
Below right: With the flesh
removed, an anatomist pulls
back the ribs with his left hand
to enable an incision from the
neck down the right side of
the cadaver.

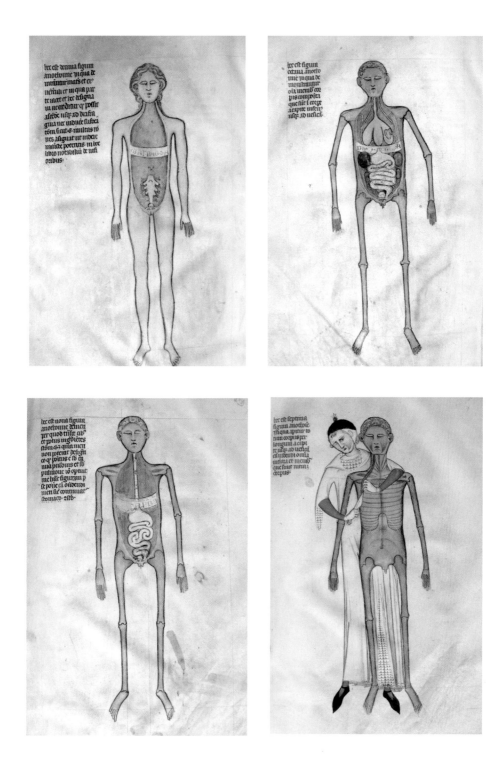

Mansur ibn Ilyas broke new ground with the innovative use of colour in anatomical diagrams. Above left: The squatting position is typical of Middle Eastern representations of anatomy, here illustrating the muscles and nervous system of a male body. Above right: The human skeleton, showing the ribs, spine and the bones of the hand and foot. Below left: The venous system, with the organs picked out in various colours of ink. Below right: Further details of the nervous system, showing pairs of nerves in different colours.

anatomist's library, *Anathomia Philippi Septimi* (*An Anatomy for Philippe VII*). (Guido's count includes an extra Philippe who co-reigned with Louis VI in the twelfth century.)

Dissection was still illegal in France in Guido's time, and his experience with Mondino in Bologna must have been invaluable, the envy of French anatomists. His book, written in 1345, may have been more widely read at first than his tutor's, whose first edition did not appear until 1475. Guido follows Mondino's method closely, following the latter's hierarchy of body parts, repeating many of the same mistakes, but correcting some, such as the shape of the spleen. It is possible that Guido acted as Mondino's *sector* on occasion, and he claims in his *Anathomia* to have undertaken many dissections himself.

His illustrations illuminate both his and Mondino's texts. They are certainly not in the same league as Leonardo da Vinci's; among his many accomplishments, Guido is no artist. His image of the removal of the cranial vault from a beheaded prisoner's skull is a disaster of perspective, like a child's drawing of an egg in an eggcup on a breakfast table. Nevertheless, it does clearly show the vault beside and not on top of the man's head, and two of the cranial sutures (the joins between the plates of the crown of the skull) are visible, like cracks in the egg. Another image shows the value of a clear diagram in conveying information, even if that information is wrong – Guido's drawing of a dissected woman shows only what he wants the viewer to see: the seven-chambered uterus which Mondino mistakenly taught his students in Bologna.

3 Mansur ibn Ilyas

The rediscovery of anatomy by Europe sometimes overshadows the continued work being done in the Islamic world. While Baghdad fell to the Mongols, other centres of learning survived; Tabriz in eastern Azerbaijan, for example. It lay on the Silk Road and benefited not only from the wealth the trade route brought but from the intellectual exchange with those passing through the city from east and west – among them Marco Polo. Tabriz was renowned especially for its collective scientific wisdom. Another city, Shiraz, was also spared by the Mongols, not once but twice, surrendering to both Genghis Khan and Tamerlane; and it developed a reputation as a centre of the arts and philosophy.

Mansur ibn Ilyas was born in Shiraz in the mid-fourteenth century to a wealthy intellectual family whose members included physicians, scholars and poets. He inherited an enquiring mind, travelled widely and made several visits to Tabriz to broaden his education and his horizons. He pursued a career as a physician and contributed an important book to the anatomist's library.

His illustrated *Tashrīḥ-i badan-i insān* (*The Anatomy of the Human Body*) is in some ways derivative – there are many references to Rhazes and Avicenna and even to the older authorities of Hippocrates and Aristotle – and most scholars agree that most of his images are copied from an earlier author. What Mansur did pioneer, however, was the use of colour in his diagrams of the organs and their vessels. Colour was frowned on at the time under Islamic teaching and Mansur's use of it was controversial. The benefit of it in clarifying visual information is, however, undeniable.

Mansur, who wisely dedicated his book to a grandson of Tamerlane, took a particular interest in foetal development. One illustration definitely attributed to him is of a

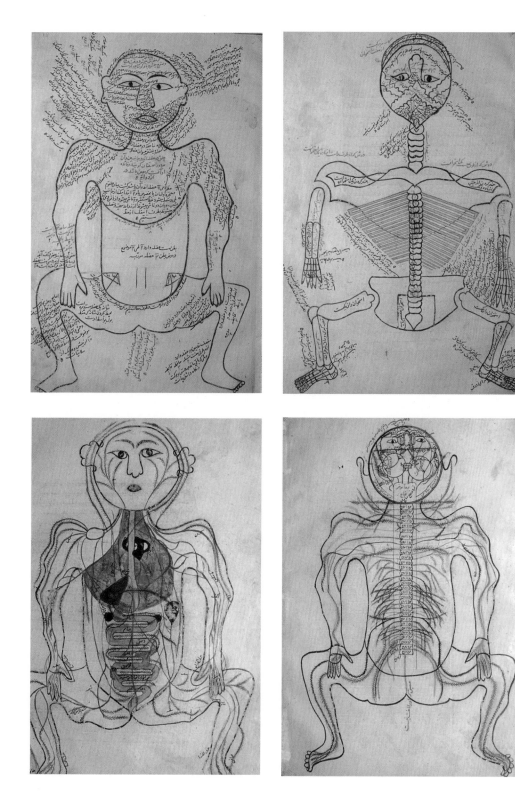

This edition of Zayn
al-Din al-Jurjani's original
work dating from 1136
opens with a double-page
illuminated introduction.

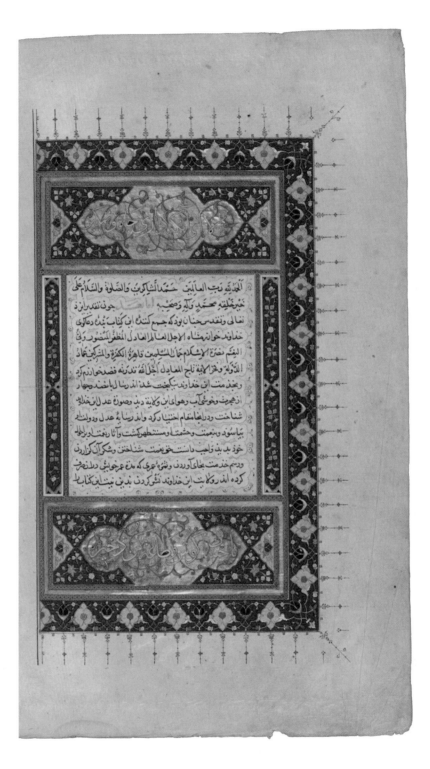

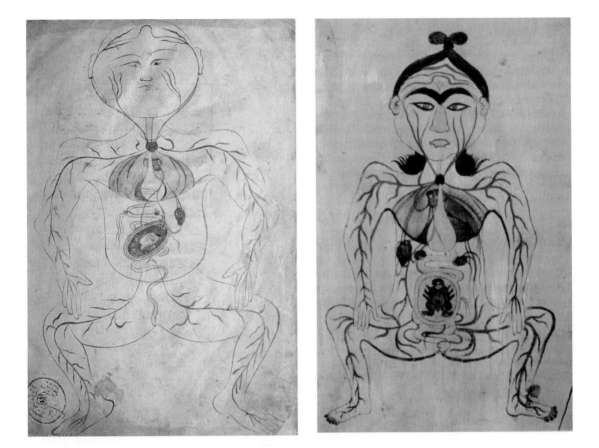

Left: Male anatomy showing the major organs. Right: Female anatomy including the womb.

pregnant woman, and he devoted an entire section to the subject. The question of whether the brain or the heart was formed first in the womb had an obvious bearing on the argument over which was the ruler of the body. Mansur reasoned the heart must come first because it contained the pneuma and heat which created and maintained the other organs. The brain was the seat of the senses; without a body made by the heart, the brain's function was redundant. Although it's a weak circular argument, Mansur was right – the heart is the first organ to be formed after conception.

The reason for doubt over some of Mansur's other illustrations is the striking similarity they bear to those of Zayn al-Jurjani, a prolific medical author working 300 years before Mansur. After a full life's study of philosophy, theology, pharmacology and medicine, Jurjani (1040–1136) was appointed physician to the court of the Shah of Khwarazm in Persia when he was in his seventies. There he wrote a medical encyclopedia, *Zakhirah-i Khwarazm Shahi* (*Thesaurus of the Shah of Khwarazm*), dedicated to his master. Jurjani made some early discoveries of the connection between goitres of the neck, palpitations and bulging eyes, which would not be rediscovered until Caleb Parry's work in the early nineteenth century. Although Jurjani's *Thesaurus* was a general work, it included a section on anatomy, greatly, but not entirely, derived from Avicenna. It was illustrated in a distinctive style, using the template of a human figure squatting in a frog-like pose over which selected anatomical details were drawn and labelled to illustrate the point being made.

Many of Mansur's illustrations adopt the same format, which – it has been argued – has its roots in an even earlier tradition, the so-called Five Pictures Series. Karl Sudhoff, a German medical historian in the early twentieth century, identified a set of five standard anatomical views which were inserted into many twelfth- and thirteenth-century manuscripts. They were crude attempts to illustrate the skeletal, nervous, muscular, venous and arterial systems, sometimes with a sixth diagram of a pregnant woman. The oldest were discovered in a Bavarian monastery among the pages of a text dated to 1158. They generally adopted the same frog-like pose, which appears to be of Persian origin and to have influenced later anatomical images from the Indian subcontinent well into the eighteenth century, where they were adapted to illustrate ayurvedic principles. The origins of the tradition are uncertain, but based on the anatomical detail and the errors contained within them they may have been early attempts to illustrate Galen, drawn by people who

The Anatomy Theatre, Bologna University

The chamber, built entirely of sprucewood, took 101 years to complete (1636–1737). Figures of the great anatomists, including Hippocrates and Galen, line the walls, and dissections here were originally conducted by candlelight.

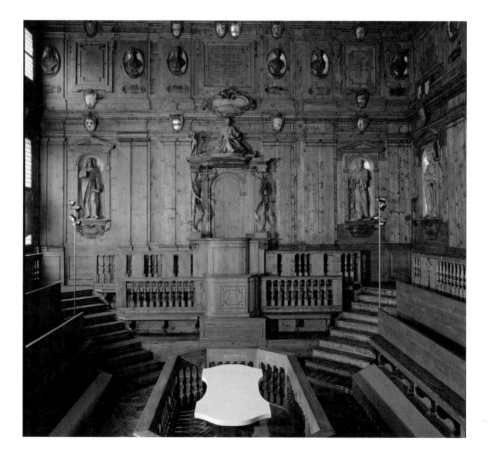

had not undertaken any dissections themselves and only had Galen's descriptions to guide them. The style of Mansur's and Jurjani's diagrams is a tantalising potential link backwards to Galen and forwards to Asian medicine, and a reminder that a Eurocentric history of anatomy does not paint the full picture.

4 Supply and demand

In fifteenth-century Europe, the legalisation of human dissections, first in Bologna and gradually in other medical schools in northern Italy, created an unforeseen problem. Dissections were carried out on the bodies of executed prisoners; but capital punishment was a rare sentence in Italy at the time. There simply weren't enough dead criminals to go round, especially at the right time of year. In a world without refrigeration, winter was the best time to study anatomy, because bodies being painstakingly dissected by inexperienced learners putrefied more slowly in the cold months. The Galenic sequence of dissection was dictated largely by the rate at which the various organs of the body deteriorated.

In the absence of the executed, students (who were obliged to attend dissections as part of their training) were reduced to procuring their own cadavers. Bodysnatching was undoubtedly one way round the problem and there is a record of the prosecution of four Bolognese students unearthing a corpse on behalf of their tutor; but for more law-abiding students there was another method. Eager learners and their teachers are known to have approached the bereaved families of recently deceased citizens, offering to pay for the funeral and to swell the ranks of mourners in return for the use of the corpse in class afterwards.

The shortage became more acute as the century progressed and the popularity of anatomy increased. That popularity was driven not only by the availability of public dissections (sufficient bodies permitting) but by a renewed interest in the art of antiquity – the graceful and anatomically correct figures of Greek and Roman sculpture. Artists sought to understand the human body so that they could accurately reproduce its movements and positions in their work. It's a nice meeting of disciplines. The Italian Renaissance, that most artistic of art movements, relied in part on that most scientific of early medical studies, anatomy.

5 Alessandro Achillini

Italy, and Bologna in particular, continued to dominate the anatomical world for the rest of the fifteenth century. Individuals made small but significant improvements to the Galenic model, which nevertheless was broadly accepted wholesale.

Alessandro Achillini (1463–1512) studied at Bologna soon after Mondino's *Anathomia corporis humani* was first published. He went on to teach at the city's university and to make several skeletal discoveries, including the malleus and the incus, two tiny bones in the inner ear. Achillini was the first to identify the seven bones which make up the tarsus – the complex part of the foot between the toes and the leg. He had a long tenure at Bologna – twenty-eight years – and his writings indicate a wealth of practical anatomical experience. He identified two areas of the brain, the fornix and the infundibulum; and the ducts which carry saliva from the glands beneath the jaw to the mouth.

Achillini demonstrated his experience in his *Annotationes anatomicae* (*Anatomical Notes*), in which he compared his own dissections to those of Galen and Avicenna, noting the similarities and differences he observed – an early but significant challenge to Galen's unquestioned supremacy. The book also contains directions for some common anatomical operations including castration and (after death) the removal of the rib cage to facilitate dissection.

He was, by all accounts, a modest man with no pretensions or ambitions – one writer described him as 'unskilled in the arts of adulation and double-dealing'. He was a popular teacher, whom his students felt able to tease while at the same time admiring him. Like many academics, he became rather rigid in his opinions but enjoyed cheerfully arguing his position with other staff members and students. He was wedded to his work and never married; nor did he publish in his lifetime. One collection his writings, *De humani corporis anatomia* (*The Anatomy of the Human Body*), was printed in Venice in 1516; and his *Annotationes anatomicae* were published in Bologna by his brother Giovanni Filoteo in 1520.

6 Antonio Benivieni

A near contemporary of Alessandro Achillini, Antonio Benivieni (1443–1502), studied medicine at the universities of Pisa and Siena. He came from a wealthy family in Florence and did not rely on medicine for his income. In that sense he was an early example of the gentleman scientist, the enthusiastic amateur on whom so much progress depended in all the sciences until the late nineteenth century.

But Benivieni was no dabbler. His brother Girolamo wrote later that Antonio had been 'medicating for about thirty-two years'. He was a very successful doctor, admired for his accurate diagnoses, his careful remedies and his surgical skill. Thanks to his social position he ministered to the highest families in the Florentine Republic, including Lorenzo the Magnificent – Lorenzo de' Medici, the ruler of the Republic. Lorenzo was a patron of many institutions in Florence, and the two men seem to have been genuine friends. Lorenzo trusted Benivieni enough to allow him to treat his daughter, and Benivieni was also physician to other noble families and institutions, including several convents in the city which were sponsored by Lorenzo. Benivieni dedicated three books to his patron: *In Praise of the Heavens*, *On a Healthy Regimen* and *On Disease*.

Lorenzo was an enthusiastic patron of the arts and a key player in the emergence of the Italian Renaissance. Benivieni's anatomical work is therefore of particular interest. In fact, it reflects a coming of age for anatomy. By the fifteenth century anatomy was indisputably a natural science, not a divine mystery or a bloodless philosophical theory – despite the persistence of belief in Galen's humors. Here were real physical organs and vessels, whose malfunctions, not merely from injury but also from disease, could cause illness and death. For curious people, autopsy was becoming a new way of establishing the cause of death. Anatomy was no longer a detached science but a tool of practical use and Antonio Benivieni is today regarded as the father of pathology. As the body of anatomical knowledge grew, Benivieni became more interested in what abnormal anatomy looked like, and what its effects were on life.

By the end of the fifteenth century, it was a relatively common practice both in hospitals and in the private homes of those who could afford one to employ a good anatomist-surgeon to perform an autopsy – and anatomists in need of bodies to dissect were only too happy to oblige. Abnormal anatomy, or teratology, spills out from the pages of Benivieni's great book *De abditis morborum causis* (*The Hidden Causes of Disease*). He describes cancers of the stomach, intestinal perforation, a peritoneal abscess, an abnormally enlarged colon and his discovery of gall bladder stones. The book also contains his pioneering study of parasitic worms and of the in-utero transfer of syphilis from mother to child. Some of his guidelines for the process of autopsy are still part of modern practice. It is a landmark publication.

Like Achillini, Benivieni did not publish in his lifetime. Under its full title, *De abditis nonnullis ac mirandis morborum et sanationum causis* (*On Some of the Hidden and Wondrous Causes of Diseases and Healing*) was dedicated to Lorenzo and only printed in 1507 after the manuscript was discovered by Girolamo sorting

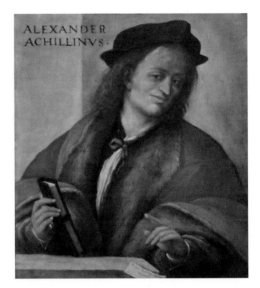

through his late brother's effects. The work, in Latin, went through many editions and, long after the original had been lost, a sixteenth-century version was the basis for a translation into Italian in the nineteenth century. The translator, Carlo Burci, then rediscovered the original manuscript during his research. It contained sections lost in the later editions, which Burci included in a later history of medicine. Burci's translations offer the most complete text we may ever have of Benivieni's groundbreaking work: the original which he found has once again been lost.

The advent of printing, like the invention of the internet, made the rapid exchange of information possible in a way that could not have been imagined beforehand. The rush of publications at the end of the fifteenth century and the beginning of the sixteenth was not confined to Italy or the Middle East. The period saw new works by several significant German authors, evidence of the spread of anatomical knowledge and curiosity to northern Europe.

7 Johannes de Ketham

Johannes de Ketham (active 1460–91) has achieved a measure of fame by association with *Fasciculus medicinae* (*Medical Anthology*), an anthology of anonymous medieval treatises published in Venice in 1491. Ketham was a German physician who practiced in Venice and Vienna, but he was not an author and probably not even an editor of the collection. He simply owned one of the two manuscripts in which the treatises were discovered.

Nevertheless, *Fasciculus medicinae* traditionally bears his name; and it is noteworthy because it was the first printed book of anatomy to contain illustrations. Only later editions of Mondino's *Anathomia* carried images. *Fasciculus medicinae* contains ten full-page woodcuts – five full-figure anatomical drawings, one chart for analysing the colour of a patient's urine and four general scenes. The scenes are a title page showing a learned man and his books; a consultation of physicians; the treatment of a patient in his

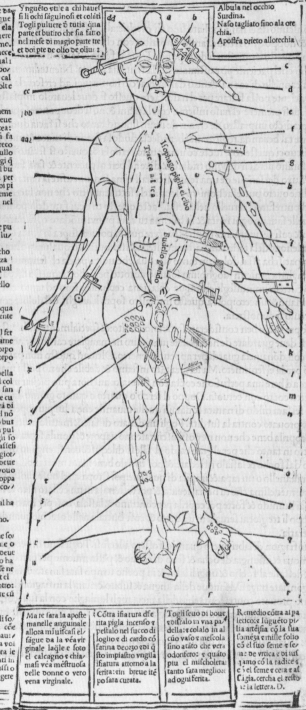

Se alcuno cascaffe da
alto et hauesse fague
pesto i dosso et o ela
to: p farlo dissoluere
et spargei nel huome.
Togli tre carboni acce
fi di ozza: et stoual e
nel vino biaco et bo
no et dalo ad bere cal
do la matia piu volte

Nota che qn vn mem
bro e tagliato se deue
curare cu la dialtea:
el ql e vnguento si fa
coi: piglia fenogreco
et seme olin e redullo
in puluere: et spargi q
sta puluef sopra el bu
tiro et laffalo cofi per
doi o tre giorni: poi pi
glia fenogreco e seme
lino Circa el resto nel
la littera. B.

Ferita che hacarne pu
tre fata intorno de lu
na parte in altra
Taglio di stomacho
di figato et de milza
Ferita fixa de la qual
e perso el coltello.
Taglio del budello
grande.

Ferita di la et di qua
ferita profondamente
fixa per tutto.
Saeta dela qual el fer
ro erimafto nela carne
roifura e tuto elcorpo
varoli p tuto el corpo

Cotra el taglio della
vena magiore nel col
lo qn no itagna el fan
gue allora se deue cu
ire la vena con gra di
ligentia tanto chel no
eichi et facto qsto but
tali sopra la ferita pul
uere roffe et poegli fo
pra epiastro: et laffefi
cofi fino alerto giot
no lo epiastro si deue
fare di chiara de vouo
con incenso et stoppa
da poi si medica co
mele ferite.
Ferita streta laqual ha
pertuto busi.
Trafixion di legno.

Cotra le feride che fo
no fate da veretoi e o
fageta: allora no deue
trare el ligno o vo ha
fta del ferro: ma se ne
vscito el legno: et el
ferro erimafto dentro:
allora si di cercare cu
la fpatula.

De varoli li quali fo
no certe vefi che cce
i pefie togliono hau
re li puti: et alcua vol
ta li vecchi ancora le
hanno: et fono fati i
doi modi cioe rossi o
biache si duemolgere

Ynguéto vtile a chi hauef
fi li ochi faguinofi et coláti
Togli puluere d tutia qua
parte et butiro che fia fato
nel mefe di magio parte tre
et doi pte di olio de oliu

Ilcophago piglia el cibo

Trac ea a£ ea

Budello grando

Albula nel occhio
Surdina.
Nafo tagliato fino ala ore
chia.
Apoftea drieto allorechia

Togli femola o
meto et cuocil
agiongi affuny
empiaftro con
ponilo sopra li
i sfiati: ma se
giouera allor
la cotega del c
guarda fe et tor
no offo di det
ito cerca nela

La poftema fu
nir e in tre luo
corpo hüano: o
le orechie coe m
lo cioe nella re
aiata: et allora i
nuifcefe la vea
lica da luno et
o accio della pte
e fi n e vechio ta
fi minuifcha el I

Taglio di vena
no itagna el fang

Trafiffion de cost
banda in banda
Taglio del budel
grande.
Trafiffion dil coltel
de bada in banda
Ferite penetrata ad
ambedoi le parte d
la e de qua.

Cotra ferita fixa o vo
profonda se la ferita
butta molto fague al
lora brufa lodice et fa
ne puluere et buitala
sopra la ferita o voto
gli qlla fubititia che
firade della charta p
gamena et ponela fo
pra tal ferita et ancora
chiara vouo et fa
impiaftro et ligalo fo
pra la ferita conftop
pa de caneua.

Apoftema nelle an
guinaglie.
Se vna ferita fiffa fara
profonda et no vicina
fangue effendo caua
to lo instrumeto allo
ra due iacere sopra la
ferita ad cio che efc i
fuora, el fangue et
imund tie: e fe in tal
modo no efcuiene de
ue fofnar tanto nel la
ferita fino a tanto ch
p quel fiato vfciran o.
Circa el refto nella lit
tera. E.
Admaturare vno apo
stema o altra infiadu
ra: Cuoci el seme lino
in buttro: et laffalo co
cere fino a tato che ba
ite: et vnguetonobi
le cotra apoftena o al
tra infiatura et cotie
quente mete ad ogni
ferita.
Cotra le veruce: piglia
sterco de cane e dilate
e tra doue ha vrina te
et falla cuocere

Ma te fara la aposte
manelle anguinale
alloza miuifcafi el
fague da la vea vir
ginale lacle e foto
el calcagno e chia
mafi vea meftruofa
delle donne o vero
vena virginale.

Cotra ifiatura dfe
rita pigla incenfo e
peftalo nel fucco di
loglio e di cardo co
farina deozzo doi q
sto impiaftro vngila
ifiatura attorno a la
ferita: in breue ité
po fara curata.

Togli feuo di boue
voftalo in vna pa
della: e colalo in al
cuo vafo e mefcola
fino atato che vera
odorifero: e quáto
piu el nifcholera
tanto fara meglio
ad ogni ferita.

Remedio cotra ai pa
letico: e lügueto pi
tia artéfia co la fua
fométa e mille folio
co el suo seme e fer
me de vrtica e di tuf
qamo co la radice e
c i el seme e cera e af
i gia. cerca el refto
ie la littera. D.

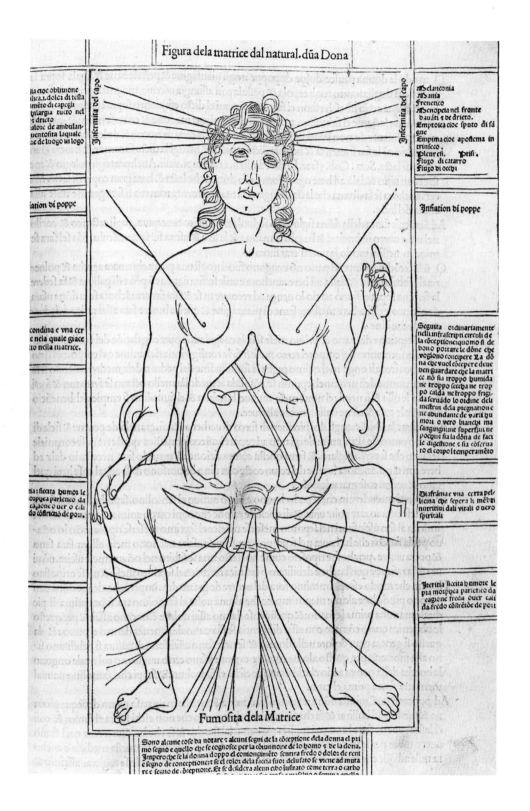

Fasciculus medicinae (1491)

An anatomy lesson under way, showing the *lector*, *sector* and *ostensor*. No one except the *sector* is paying much attention to the cadaver, below which a basket lies ready to receive discarded flesh and organs.

The Reward of Cruelty (1751)

The fourth plate in William Hogarth's series *The Four Stages of Cruelty* elaborates on the illustration of an anatomy lesson in Johannes de Ketham's *Fasciculus medicinae* with additional amusing details like the scavenging dog and the boiling pot of bones.

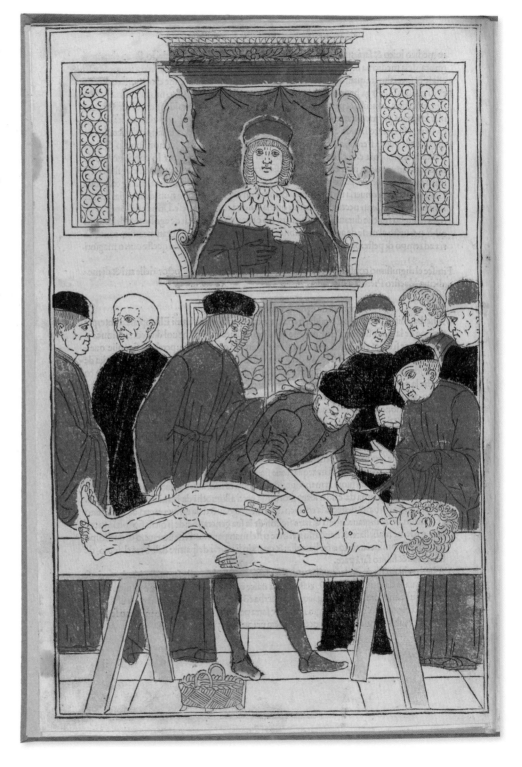

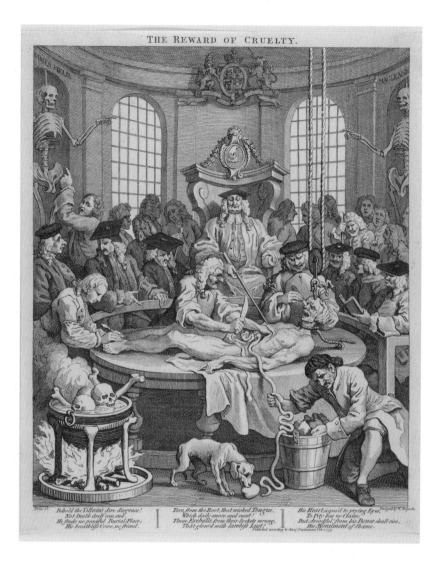

bed; and a public dissection underway, complete with *lector*, *sector* and *ostensor*. The figures are naturalistic and not at all frog-like: the Renaissance was by now well underway.

There are some nice details in the pictures: a broken window behind the *lector* and a basket on the floor, presumably to receive discarded organs. In another, the bedridden patient is attended not only by a physician taking his pulse but also by a cat. Ketham's book went through several editions, including an Italian translation in 1495; and it appears to have been familiar to readers in the mid-eighteenth century, when the last plate of William Hogarth's series *The Four Stages of Cruelty* (1751) was clearly based on the Ketham image of a public dissection.

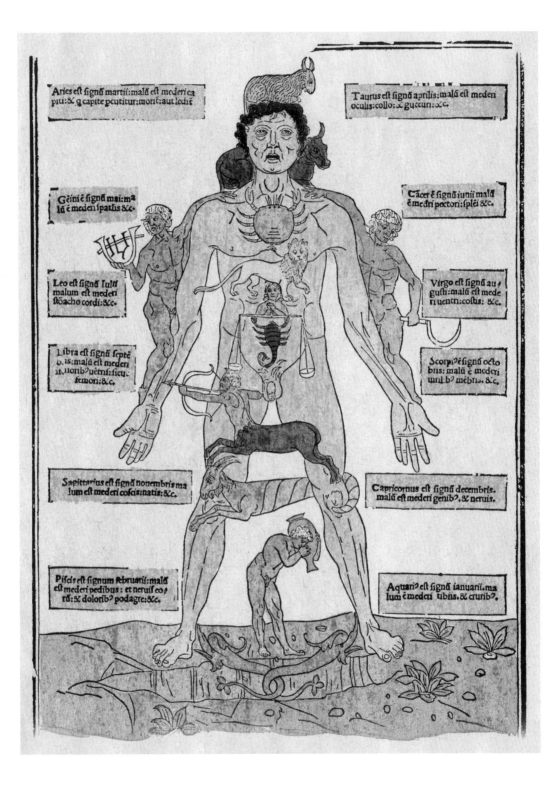

8 Hieronymus Brunschwig

Another German, Hieronymus Brunschwig (1450–1512) from Strasbourg, wrote and published prolifically during his life, and his *Liber de arte distillandi de compositis* (*Book on the Art of Compound Distilling*), published in the year of his death was a final exposition of his ideas. It was a technical manual for preparing simple (single-ingredient) and compound medicines through distillation, filtration and diffusion. It was effectively an elaborate herbal, expanded – in tune with the times – by anatomical illustrations of the affected parts to be treated. Brunschwig combined his knowledge of botany and alchemy with his experience as a surgeon.

His view of anatomy is important to historians because he was, according to some biographers, the first German (ahead of Ketham) to absorb Italian sources of anatomical knowledge. He claimed in his 1497 publication *Das Buch der Cirurgia* (*The Book of Surgery*) to have studied at the three greatest anatomy schools of the age – Bologna, Padua and Paris – although there is no other evidence for this. In the main he perpetuates Galen's humors and regards his concoctions as means of restoring imbalances of the humors within the body. He wrote that he had served in the Burgundian Wars of the 1470s (another unsubstantiated claim) and much of his *Cirurgia* (written not in Latin but in his native German) is concerned with healing injuries sustained on the battlefield, including bullet wounds. In German he was a *Wundarzt* – a wound doctor.

The illustrations are elaborate woodcuts of scenes, rather than strictly anatomical images. Like in *Fasciculus medicinae*, there are pictures of a consultation with physicians (in *Cirurgia* there is a man with an arrow through his forearm); of a bedridden patient; of one unfortunate man pierced through with swords and arrows and beset by clubs to the head and body, studied by some amused and dispassionate doctors. There is some anatomical detail in these scenes, but not as diagrams. Nevertheless Brunschwig's two books remained authoritative works for most of the sixteenth century – and not just in German-speaking lands. *Cirurgia* was translated into Dutch in 1517, into English in 1527, and (as evidence of its longevity) into Czech at the ancient University of Olomouc in 1559. Having brought Italian thinking to Germany, Brunschwig was a vital link in spreading it further abroad.

OPPOSITE

Fasciculus medicinae (1491)

A chart showing points for bloodletting and relating them to the signs of the Zodiac.

BELOW

Das Buch der Cirurgia (1497)

An array of surgical instruments, in a woodcut from Hieronymus Brunschwig's book, which helped spread the study of anatomy through Europe.

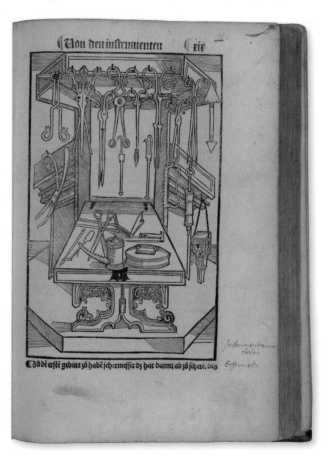

RIGHT

Das Pestbuch (1500)

The treatment of a patient suffering from the Black Death, in *Das Pestbuch* (*The Plague Book*) by Hieronymus Brunschwig. The woodcut was reused from Brunschwig's *Liber de arte distillandi de compositis* (*Book on the Art of Compound Distilling*).

OPPOSITE

Das Buch der Cirurgia (1497)

Hieronymus Brunschwig's version of the standard Wound Man illustration.

OVERLEAF

Liber de arte distillandi de simplicibus (1500)

An apothecary teaches his art, pointing to jars labelled with alchemical and hermetic symbols, in a woodcut from Hieronymus Brunschwig's *Book on the Art of Simple Distilling*.

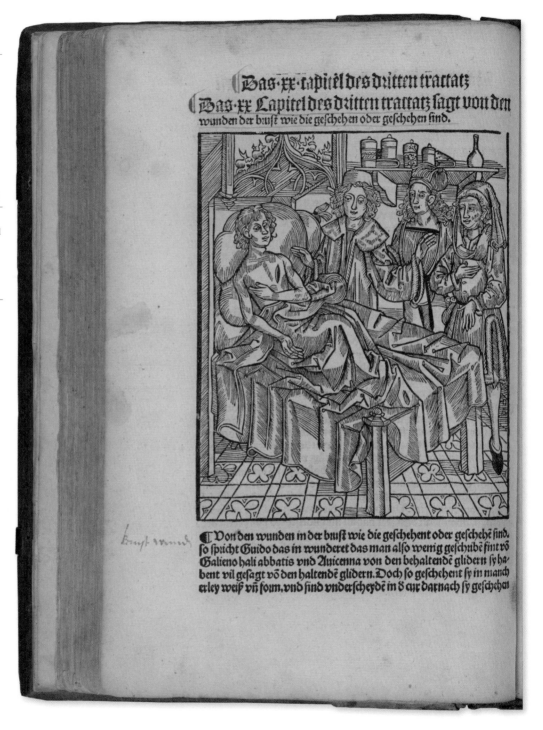

¶ Das erst capitel des andern tractat ¶ xviii

¶ Nach dem ich mit hilff des allmechtigē gotes vol
bꝛacht han disen ersten tractat. Rieff ich an sein eingebornen sun ihm̄ cri
stum sein barmherẓikeyt mir ẓů verleihen disen andern tractat ẓů mach
en alle wunden in einer gemeinen lere wie die geschehen ẓů heylen vnd ẓů
curieren.

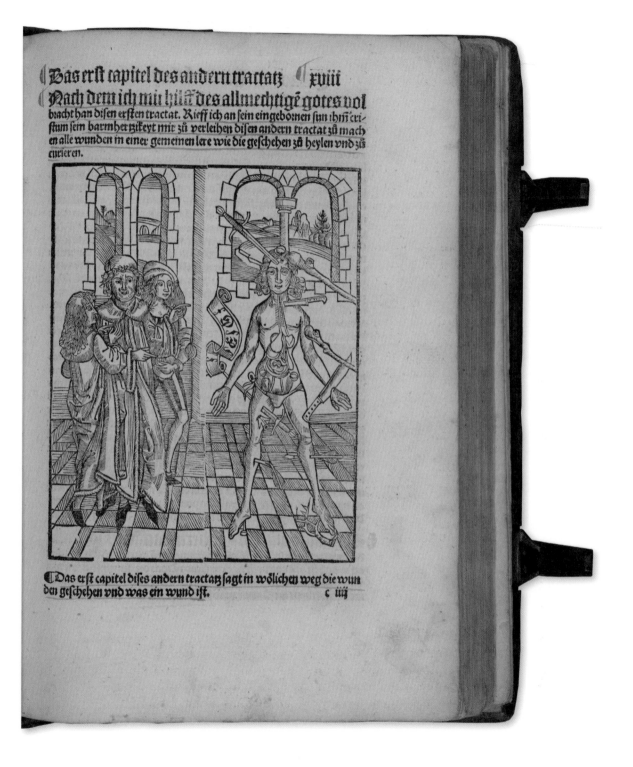

¶ Das erst capitel dises andern tractatz sagt in wōlichen weg die wun
den geschehen vnd was ein wund ist.   c iiij

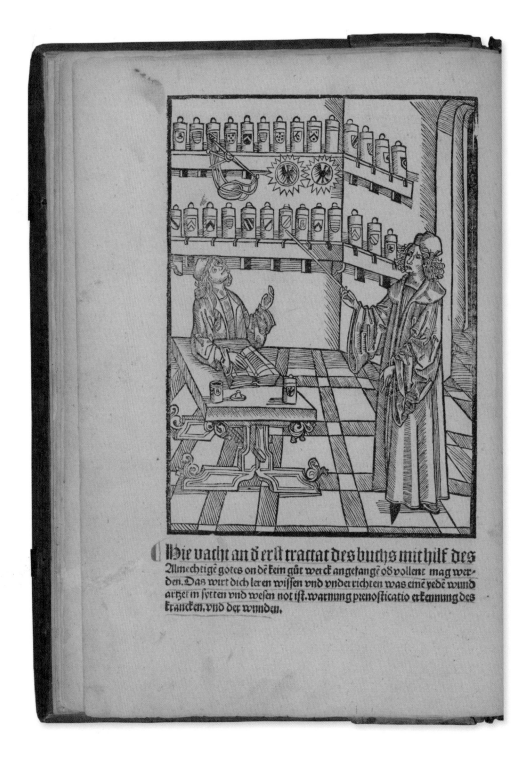

Wie vacht an d̃ erst tractat des buchs mit hilf des
Almechtigẽ gotes on dẽ kein gũt werck angefangẽ od vollent mag wer-
den. Das wirt dich leren wissen vnd vnder richten was einẽ yedẽ wund
artzet in sytten vnd wesen not ist. warnung prenosticatio erkennung des
krancken. vnd der wunden.

9 Magnus Hundt

At the very start of the sixteenth century a new German anatomy was published which gave a comprehensive picture of the sum of anatomical knowledge to date. Magnus Hundt (1449–1519) was rector of the University of Leipzig, his alma mater, and his *Antropologium de hominis dignitate, natura, et proprietatibus de elementis* (*Anthropology of the Dignity of Man, Nature and Properties, of the Elements, Parts and Members of the Human Body*) appeared in print in 1501.

Magnus Hundt also held a chair in theology at Leipzig. Beside anatomy he wrote biblical commentaries, philosophical treatises and a book of the rules of grammar. His *Antropologium* included seventeen woodcuts, and they suggest that, despite a mere ten-year gap between Ketham and Hundt, illustrators were already learning what worked and what didn't. Hundt's pictures have perspective, depth, economy and boldness of line.

They are focussed too; there are close-ups of the head, the hand, the torso and of several individual organs. It was an appropriately ambitious work for a new century. Some of the smaller diagrams were re-used from an earlier work by a colleague of Hundt's in Leipzig's Faculty of the Arts. *Compendium philosophiae naturalis* (*Compendium of Natural Philosophy*) by Johann Peyligk (1474–1522) may have been the first book to introduce new, more realistic diagrams of anatomical detail, on which Hundt built; but Peyligk's illustration of the contents of the torso is low on information compared to Hundt's.

BELOW LEFT

Compendium philosophiae naturalis (1499)

Johann Peyligk was the first anatomist to illustrate individual parts of the body in detail, although he retained many persistent fallacies such as the ventricles of the brain and the five-lobed liver, here shown gripping the stomach.

BELOW RIGHT

Antropologium de hominis dignitate, natura, et proprietatibus de elementis (1501)

Magnus Hundt built on Peyligk's innovation with greater detail, clarity and perspective.

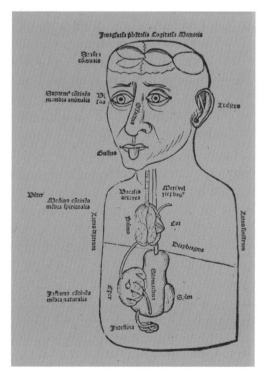

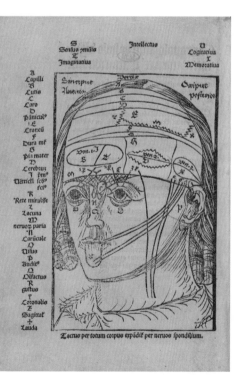

Antropologium de hominis dignitate, natura, et proprietatibus de elementis (1501)

Above left: Muscles of the male anatomy, in a bold, confident woodcut. Above right: The palm of the hand, with astrological signs for the practice of cheiromancy. Some editions of Magnus Hundt's work were hand-coloured. Below left: Internal organs of the male torso, with some indication of the sequence of dissection which revealed them. Below right: Magnus Hundt's understanding of the heart's place in the circulatory system.

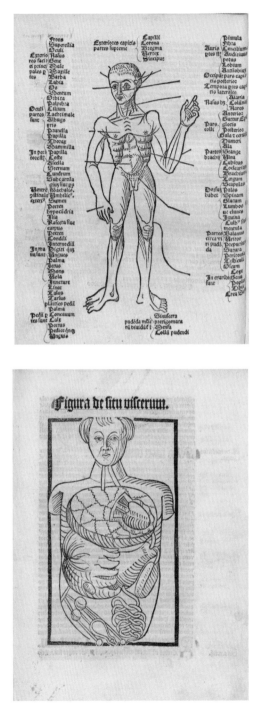

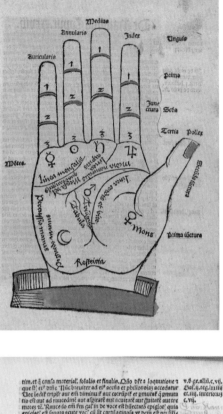

10 Gregor Reisch

Hundt aimed to explain the human body in terms of philosophy and theology as well as by its physiology. His *Antropologium* makes for a good report on the state of all those disciplines at the start of the century. Coincidentally he also coined the word 'anthropology', although not with its modern meaning. Hot on Hundt's heels came Gregor Reisch's *Margarita philosophica* (*A Philosophical Pearl*), printed in Strasbourg in 1503. Reisch (1467–1525) was a Carthusian monk who studied and taught at the University of Freiburg. What Hundt did for anatomy, Reisch attempted to do for the whole university curriculum (including anatomy) – *Margarita philosophica* was one of the very first encyclopedias of general knowledge, and so successful that it became a prescribed text in some universities for the whole of the sixteenth century, running to at least twelve editions. Copies reached Burgos in Spain and Oxford and Cambridge in England.

The book is lavishly illustrated with woodcuts. For once we know the name of the artist – Alban Graf from University of Basel – who is creditworthy for having insisted on reading the book before supplying the illustrations. The anatomy chapter includes a detailed cross-section of the eye and a diagram of the organs in situ within a dissected body.

As a theologian and philosopher Reisch drew heavily on classical thought, not only for its wisdom but the format of the book. It reads as a conversation between student and master, with questions and answers. It was intended to be read through from start to finish, not dipped into for particular topics, although it does have a list of contents and an index – then a novelty in books. The authorities invoked to answer a student's enquiry include Aristotle, Plato, Euclid, Virgil and, of course, the Bible, and the early Christian philosophers Gregory, Jerome, Ambrose and Augustine. Reisch called on more modern thinkers too: Duns Scotus, John Peckham and Peter Lombard, among them. Reisch was regarded as one of the great intellectuals of his age, and his accessible pearls of wisdom made a significant contribution to the spread of knowledge in the sixteenth century, and to the anatomist's library.

BELOW

Margarita philosophica (1503)

Gregor Reisch's attempt to encompass all knowledge in his book included this astrological guide to the human anatomy, from Pisces governing the feet to the influence of Aries on the brain.

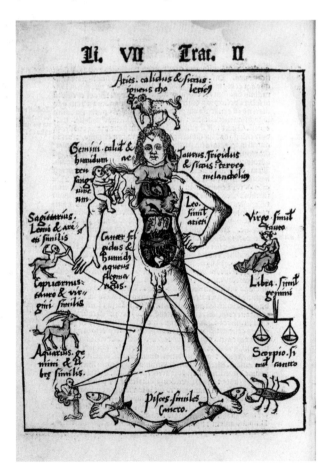

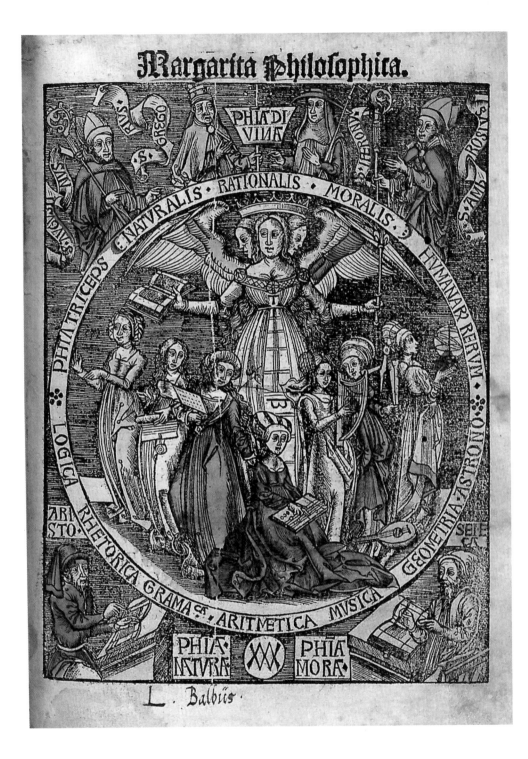

The Allegory of Philosophy
illustrates Gregor Reisch's
ambition to encompass
all strands of knowledge
– astronomy, geometry,
music, arithmetic, grammar,
rhetoric and logic – in one
comprehensive encyclopedia.
Reisch's illustrator was the
gifted Alban Graf of Basel.

A diagram of the human
eye (left), and of the brain
(right), the latter showing the
ventricles where the various
faculties of the soul were
believed to reside.

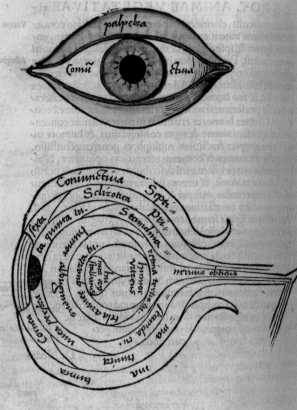

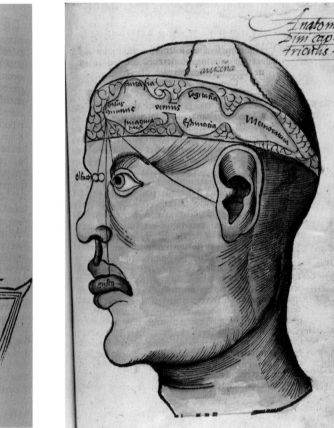

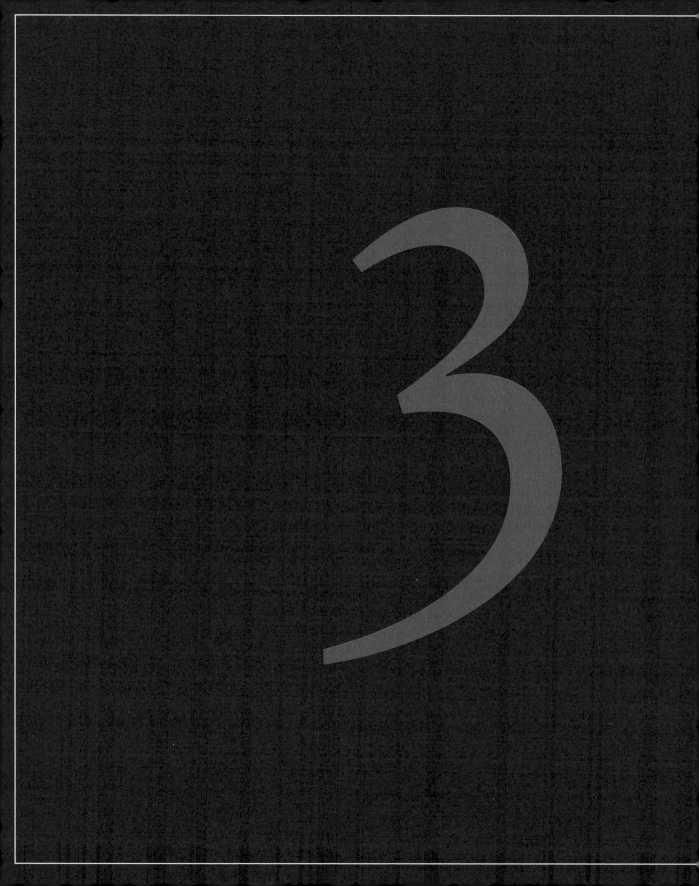

ANATOMY IN
THE RENAISSANCE
1501–1600

The sixteenth century was a dizzying time for man's understanding of the human body. The Italian Renaissance was at its creative and intellectual peak and the period produced both artistic and medical masterpieces of anatomy.

1 Berengario da Carpi

Among those who studied Mondinian anatomy in Bologna was Berengario da Carpi. He won his degree from that university in 1489, not long after the first edition of Mondino's work was published. Jacopo Berengario (*c*.1460–1530) was the son of a surgeon and had already acquired a wealth of experience at his father's side before he arrived in Bologna.

After his qualification he followed in Galen's footsteps by moving to Rome in 1494 in search of fame and fortune. He found both, thanks to an epidemic of syphilis which he was able to treat in its early stages with doses of mercury. Like Galen, his success aroused jealousy, but with his reputation established he returned to Bologna to take up a post as *Maestro nello Studio* (master of study, akin to a professorship today).

BELOW
Isagoge breves (1522)

Left: A figure in the process of shedding his skin displays not only the core muscle groups but the direction of their fibres. Right: Berengario's lifelike figures seem to be undressing willingly for the reader.

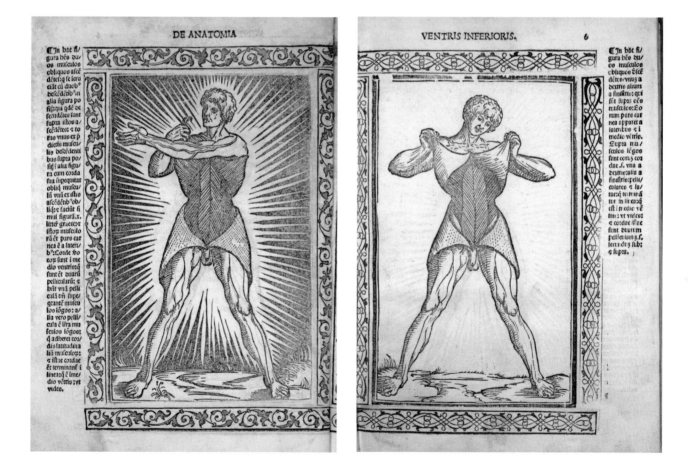

Before turning to medicine, Berengario spent time studying under the printer Aldo Manuzio who was tutor to the Prince of Carpi. With a grasp of and an interest in publishing, Berengario prepared a new edition of Mondino's *Anathomia* in 1514, and a further edition in 1521 which included his own commentary on the original. The following year he published his best-known work, *Isagoge breves perlucide ac uberime in anatomiam humani corporis* (*A Brief Introduction, Clear and Comprehensive, to the Anatomy of the Human Body*).

Isagoge breves was based, Berengario claimed, on the hundreds of dissections he had conducted. In it he was bold enough to question the infallibility of Galen, and argued for trusting one's own senses of sight, touch and smell instead of slavishly accepting the text-based wisdom of others. Based on his own dissections, he disproved the supposed existence in humans of the rete mirabile, a dense network of blood vessels which conserve heat through exchange between arteries and veins. It occurs in many vertebrates, including birds, fish and mammals, and Galen assumed it was present in human anatomy, based on his dissection of a sheep. It is not.

BELOW

Isagoge breves (1522)

Left: Berengario's figures stand astride a Renaissance landscape like Colossi, revealing their intimate abdominal secrets Right: An incision in the belly of a sleeping woman uncovers her reproductive organs.

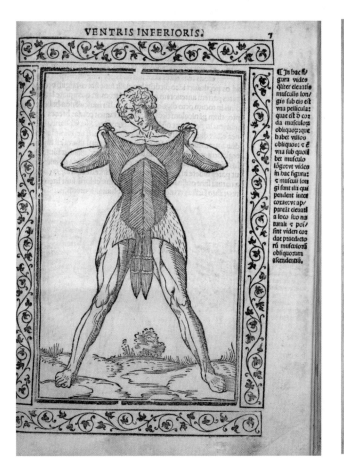

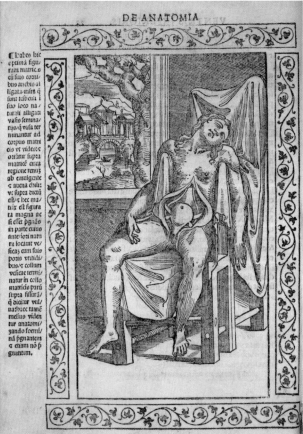

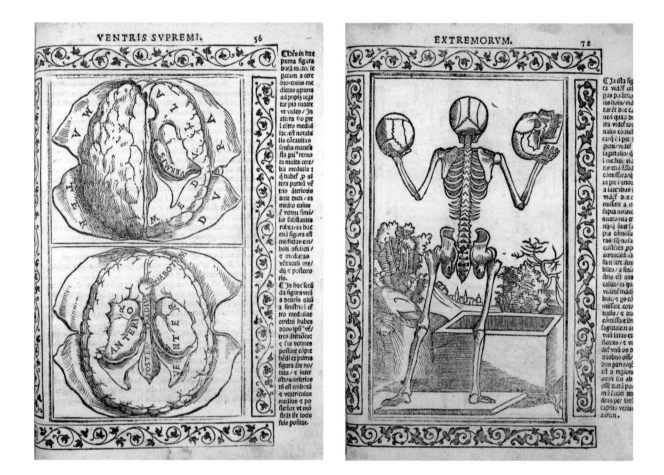

ABOVE
Isagoge breves (1522)

Left: With the scalp peeled
back, the ventricles of the brain
are uncovered in two stages.
Right: A rear view of the
human skeleton, which holds
two further views of its skull –
from above, and from the side.

2 Hans von Gersdorff

Isagoge breves is sometimes credited with being the first anatomy to include illustrations
linked to the text, although other titles might claim that achievement. Hans von
Gersdorff, for example, was – like Hieronymus Brunschwig – a *wundarzt*, a field doctor
specialising in wartime injuries. Like Brunschwig, he hailed from Strasbourg; and in
1517, only five years after Brunschwig's manual of surgical techniques, von Gersdorff
(1455–1529) published his own *Feldbuch der Wundartzney* (*Field Book of Surgery*). It is
lavishly and gruesomely illustrated with woodcuts amplifying his instructions for carrying
out an amputation or drilling into a skull. There are labelled anatomical diagrams of the
skeleton and the torso, and a wounded man being assailed by everything from a claw
hammer to a cannonball. The title page of the 1526 edition, in red and black, shows a
field doctor and his assistant treating a bleeding head wound during the siege of a city.
The blocks were probably cut by Hans Wechtlin (active 1502–26), a contemporary of the
great Renaissance woodcut artist Albrecht Dürer.

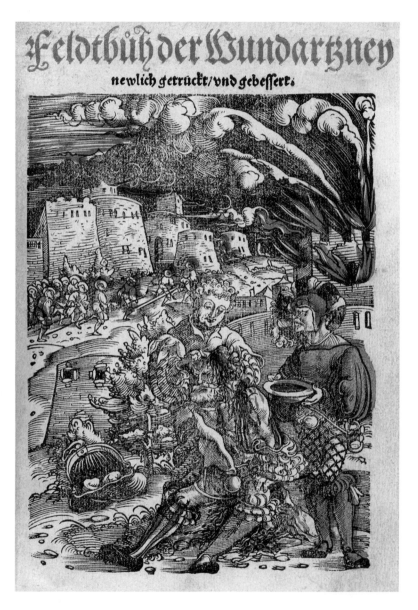

Feldbuch der
Wundartzney (1517)

A diagram of points for
bloodletting also shows
internal organs, including
those visible once the intestines
have been pulled aside.

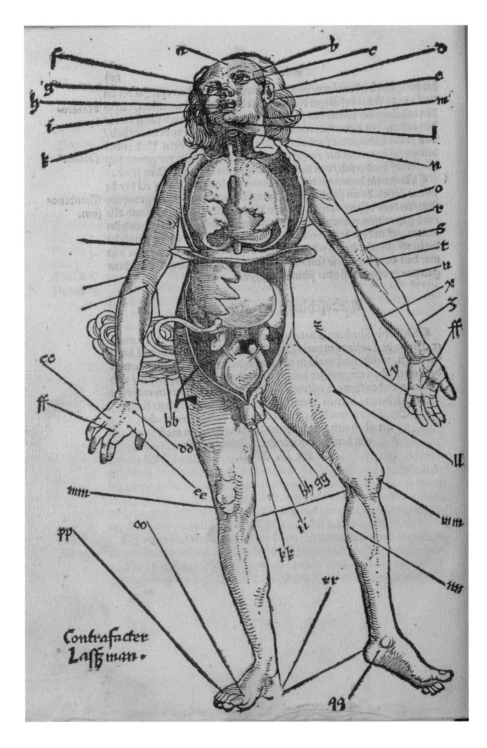

Contrafacter
Laßman.

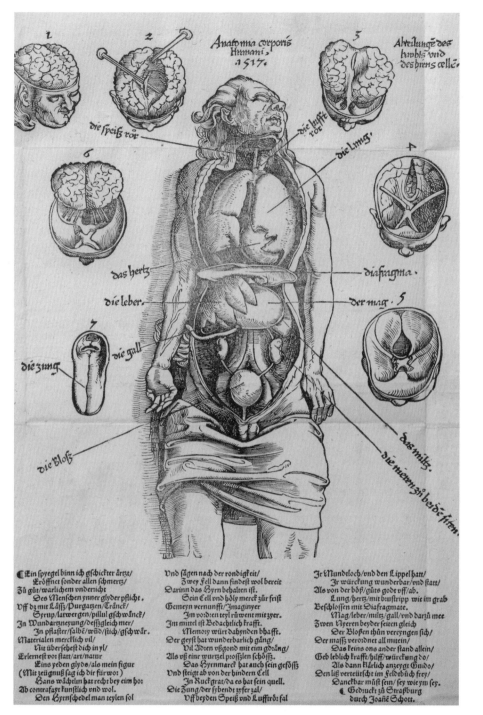

LEFT

Feldbuch der Wundartzney (1517)

Lungs, heart, five-lobed liver, stomach and bladder are all on show in this diagram, accompanied by detailed illustrations of the brain and tongue.

Feldbuch der Wundartzney (1517)

Hans von Gersdorff's woodcuts were probably carved by a contemporary of Albrecht Dürer, Hans Wechtlin. Above left: Von Gersdorff's graphic version of the standard Wound Man image. Above right: A detailed and comprehensively labelled image of the male skeleton. Below left: Cauterising a thigh injury with an iron instrument heated in a brazier stops the bleeding and sterilises the wound. Below right: A disturbing device for removing fragments of bone after a skull fracture.

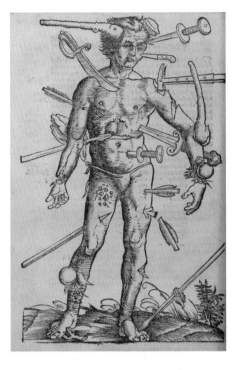
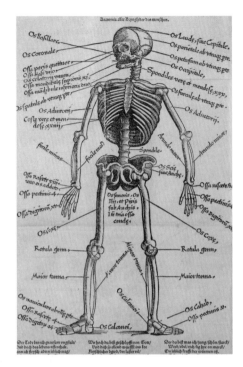
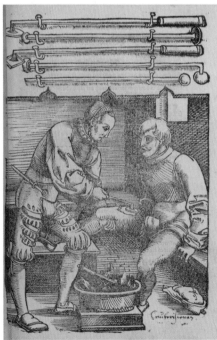
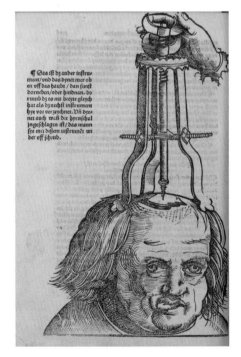

3 Leon Battista Alberti and the Pollaiuolo brothers

While anatomists pursued scientific truths about the systems and organs of the body, artists sought authenticity of portrayal. The painters and sculptors of the Renaissance were fascinated by anatomy for the impact it had on the outer appearance of human figures. By understanding the arrangement of muscles in the arm for example, they felt better able to paint a gesture; a knowledge of the skeleton contributed to realistic poses in dramatic scenes.

Artists were becoming more interested in human figures, not only those of conventional religious icons. Now they were depicting real people at work, at play, in life and in death. Because artists were concerned with appearance rather than abstract or philosophical truth, they were sometimes more observant than anatomists, and they certainly looked at the human body differently. Leon Battista Alberti (1404–72), a Genoan polymath and precursor of Leonardo da Vinci, urged his painting students, when depicting the nude, to picture the muscles and bones first and then to draw them clad in skin.

Others went further, painting or sculpting human figures, alive or dead, without the skin – in other words, flayed. Antonio del Pollaiuolo (*c*.1433–98) is known to have flayed and dissected corpses with his brother Piero (1443–96). Both were painters, working in Florence; and Antonio was also a sculptor who designed the tombs for two popes – Sixtus IV and Innocent VIII. Both brothers' work shows the influence of anatomical knowledge. Antonio's output is often characterised by a level of violence and brutality, with depictions of the body under stress. His painting of Saint Sebastian, who was martyred after being tied to a tree and shot through with arrows, is notable for including the saint's persecutors in aggressive poses; and his most famous engraving is *Battle of the Nude Men*, an exercise in drawing ten naked warriors in muscular detail, attacking or being attacked with swords, daggers, arrows and axes.

An understanding of anatomy shaped art from the mid-fifteenth century onwards. One of Antonio del Pollaiuolo's students was the painter of *The Birth of Venus*, Sandro Botticelli. It's no coincidence that three of the greatest Renaissance artists were producing their best work around the turn of the century, and all were fascinated by anatomy.

4 Leonardo da Vinci

The greatest of them all bought his first skull in 1489 and conducted his first human dissection in 1507. He was then over fifty and his subject was a 100-year-old man whose natural, peaceful death from old age Da Vinci (1452–1519) had just witnessed. His efforts with a scalpel, guided

BELOW

The Martyrdom of St Sebastian (1475)

Antonio del Pollaiuolo's painting is typical of many such images of the period which took the opportunity to display aggression and tension under the guise of religious imagery.

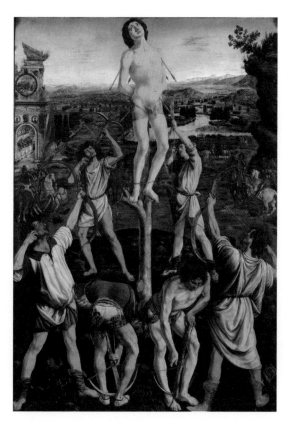

***Battle of the Nude
Men (c.1465)***

This engraving by Antonio
del Pollaiuolo is a showcase
for his understanding of
muscular anatomy, which he
acquired by conducting his
own dissections.

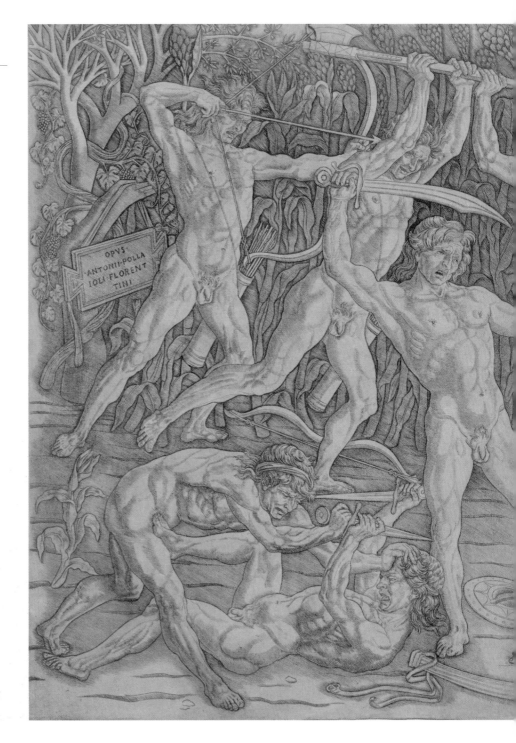

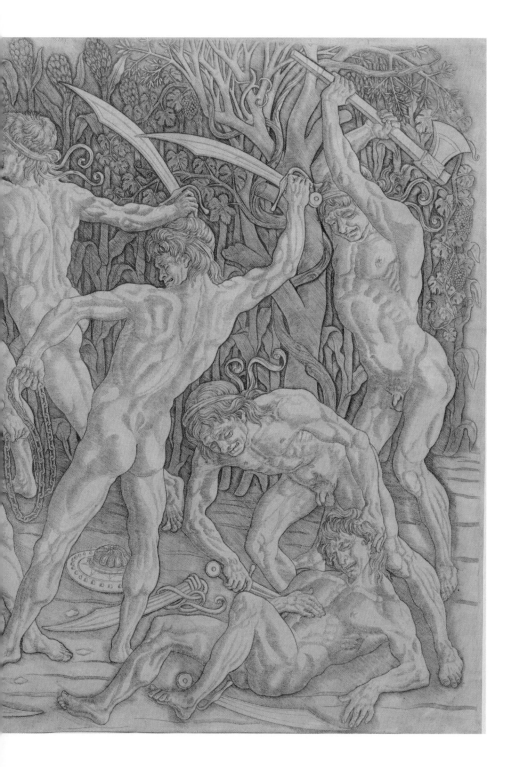

OPPOSITE
Leonardo da Vinci

Study of the foetus in the
womb. Da Vinci's advanced
anatomical drawings remained
hidden for almost 400 years
after his death.

by the anatomist Marcantonio della Torre (1481–1511), were at first clouded by a traditional view of anatomy. Della Torre lectured at the Universities of Padua and Pavia and may have published his own anatomical texts, although none survive. Historians believe he and da Vinci intended to write a book together, and over the next five years da Vinci produced a portfolio of more than 750 anatomical drawings, the like of which had never been seen before. His draughtsmanship is exquisite.

The painter of the *Mona Lisa* and designer of a helicopter was a competent anatomist too. His sketches are magnificently accurate, implying a sharp eye and a steady hand in the race to observe and record before decomposition set in. Many of them were drawn over the winter of 1510–11 with della Torre in Pavia.

In da Vinci's familiar mirror-written notes alongside his drawings, it's clear that he struggled at first with the received wisdom of anatomy – what he'd been told he would see – compared to his own explanations for what he was uncovering. For example, was the heart the source of pneuma, that 'noble spirit', as della Torre insisted? Or was it what da Vinci saw, a muscle pumping blood around the body?

Della Torre's death in 1511 put an end to the joint project and da Vinci moved into the Villa Melzi, east of Milan. There, still curious about anatomy but without access to the human bodies acquired by della Torre, he dissected birds and animals. From an ox heart he was able finally to confirm that the heart, not the liver, was central to the blood system. He even made a glass model of the aorta to study the flow through it, adding grass seeds to water to make the flow visible. In this work he was agonisingly close to making the breakthrough discovery of blood circulation which the English anatomist William Harvey finally achieved 120 years later.

Da Vinci made discoveries in the brain too. He took wax casts of the cerebral ventricles, and proved that no humors resided there, as traditional anatomy insisted. He was the first to describe atherosclerosis, the build-up of lesions on artery walls which can lead to a narrowing of the arteries, a condition which contributed to the death of his centenarian in 1507. The old man had cirrhosis of the liver, which da Vinci also described for the first time. His was the first correct study of the spine and the engineer in him was fascinated by the musculature of the skeleton; 'But how does it work?', he asked himself in one of his notes. Many of his drawings are studies in biomechanics; and relatively few are of internal organs such as the spleen, liver and kidney, which are among the first things to decompose after death.

By 1513 he was living in Rome and, with the help of the Spirito Santo hospital, dissecting human cadavers again. Although the Church did not oppose anatomy, da Vinci was reported to the Vatican by a German maker of mirrors who objected to the practice; and Pope Leo X ordered him to stop. When France conquered Milan in 1515, the French king Francis I became da Vinci's new patron and installed him in the Chateau d'Amboise on the River Loire. Leonardo remained inventive until the end, designing a mechanical lion which walked towards the king and opened up at the touch of a wand to reveal lily flowers, the fleurs-de-lys which were the royal symbol. But he suffered a series of strokes which paralysed his right arm and put an end to his anatomical exploration.

After da Vinci's death, from another stroke in 1519, his anatomy drawings passed to his apprentice Francesco Melzi (who had grown up in the villa east of Milan in which da

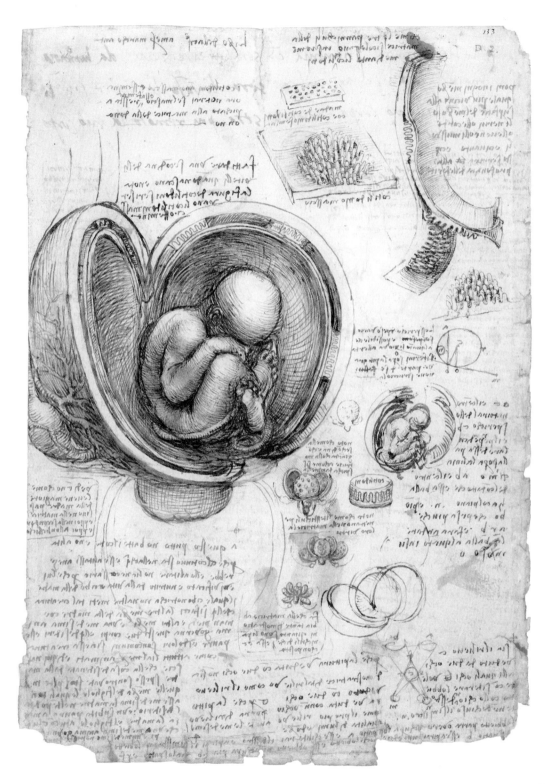

Leonardo da Vinci

The principal organs and cardiovascular system of the female anatomy. Da Vinci brought art techniques to his anatomy drawings, using light and shade, colour washes and different shades of chalk.

Leonardo da Vinci

Above left: Skeletal studies of the spine and thorax from the neck to the pelvis, and of a right leg. Above right: Two views of the skull. Da Vinci's observation of detail was unparalleled. In the upper image for example, the dot on the cheekbone is the zygomaticofacial foramen, through which facial nerves pass. Below left: Proportional study of a man in profile. The grid on the man's face shows Da Vinci's scientific, mathematical approach to art. This well-used page also contains sketches of men on horseback. Below right: The gastrointestinal tract, beside diagrams of the ureterovesical valve (above) and of bladders (below). In his notes Da Vinci challenges the dominant view of the flow of urine, which held that the valve closed under pressure from a full bladder.

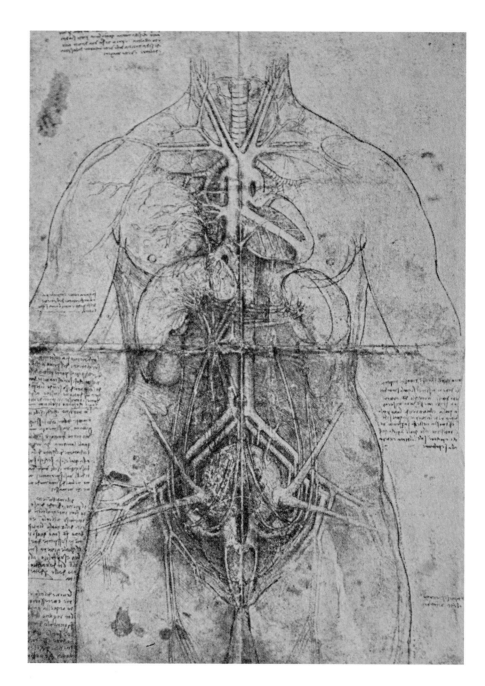

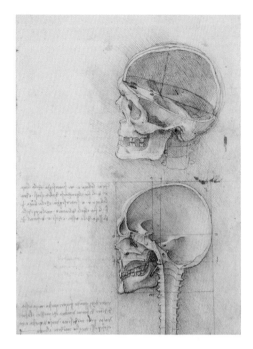

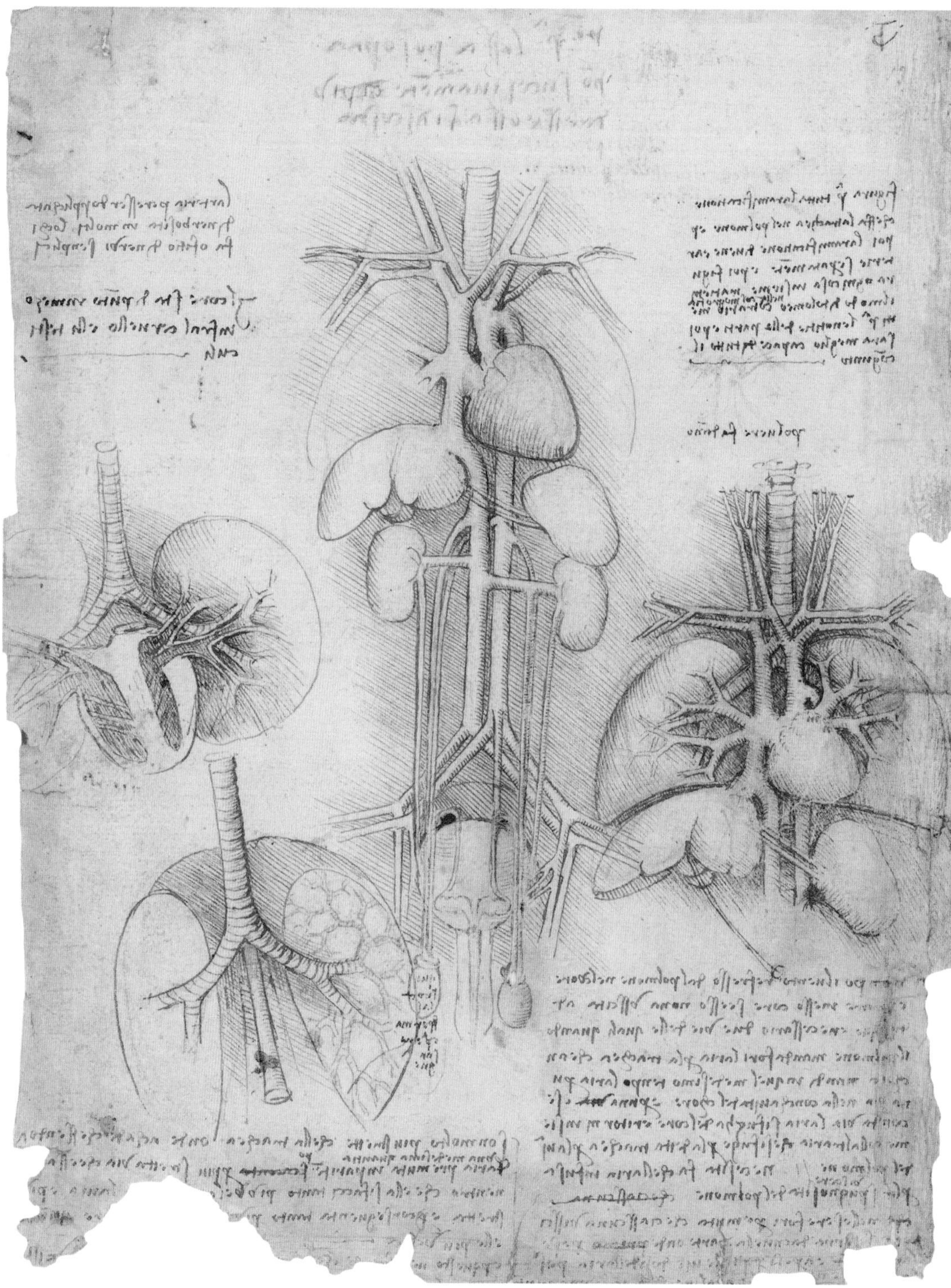

Vinci lived). After Melzi's death in 1570 the drawings were bought by Pompeo Leoni, a sculptor working for the king of Spain. By 1630 they were the property of England's Earl of Arundel, Thomas Howard; and by 1690 he had either sold or donated them to William and Mary, the king and queen of England. They remain in the British royal art collection today.

Leonardo da Vinci's enthusiasm for anatomy was intense. It's interesting that it developed late in the life of a man who had already demonstrated a superhuman grasp of so many fields of endeavour. Perhaps he sensed his own mortality; or perhaps he was simply in tune with his Renaissance times. That he never published his studies and observations was a huge loss to the science of anatomy, which had to wait centuries to make the same discoveries. Any book by da Vinci in the anatomist's library would be a recent addition; his drawings finally made it into print in 1900.

5 Albrecht Dürer

The publications of Johannes de Ketham, Hieronymus Brunschwig, Magnus Hundt, Gregor Reisch and others were instrumental in sparking the so-called Northern Renaissance in Germany and the Netherlands. Albrecht Dürer (1471–1528), who lived and worked in Nuremburg (then an imperial city of the Holy Roman Empire), made two artistic pilgrimages to northern Italy which had a profound impact on his work. He visited Padua, Mantua and Venice and absorbed the influence of Antonio del Pollaiuolo, Giovanni Bellini and Andrea Mantegna, among others. He made and printed copies of the latter's work, and in one of his sketchbooks he copied one of Leonardo da Vinci's drawings of an arm. He must therefore have seen some of da Vinci's anatomies first-hand, and perhaps met the great man himself.

As printing spread, so it drew attention to the craft of the woodcut image. Dürer, a modern man, was apprenticed to Michael Wolgemut, a woodcutter and artist in Nuremberg, which was emerging as a centre of publishing. Dürer's godfather was the most successful printer in Germany at the time and his father was a goldsmith from whom Dürer acquired both business sense and an interest in engraving. Throughout his life, he made more money from selling prints of his woodcuts and engravings than from painting.

It's uncertain whether Dürer ever attended or conducted a dissection. It was an essential part of an artist's training, but not of a woodcutter's. But his interest in it is undeniable. His two portraits of Adam and Eve, an engraving from 1504 and a painting from 1507, demonstrate his grasp of anatomy and the influence of the Italian journey he made between the two. The first demonstrates his skill as an engraver in a densely detailed work of which he was so proud that he added not only his full name but the address (his own) from which admirers could buy copies. The second strips out all extraneous detail to concentrate on the figures, which are the first full-size naked portraits ever produced in Germany.

If his Adams and Eves are anatomically idealised, his contribution to the library is not. Albrecht Dürer's *Vier Bücher von menschlicher Proportion* (*Four Books on Human Proportion*) was published in 1528, six months after his death. He had been writing it since 1512 and completed it in 1528, not long before his died. The original manuscript of the first volume survives, with Dürer's note on the title page: '1523 at Nuremberg, this

Adam and Eve (1504, 1507)

Albrecht Dürer's two images of
Adam and Eve were made only
three years apart but illustrate
the influence of a journey to
Italy which he made between
the two.

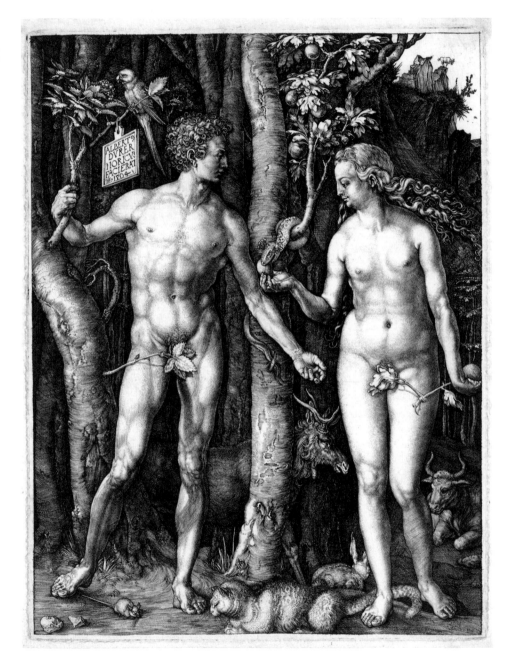

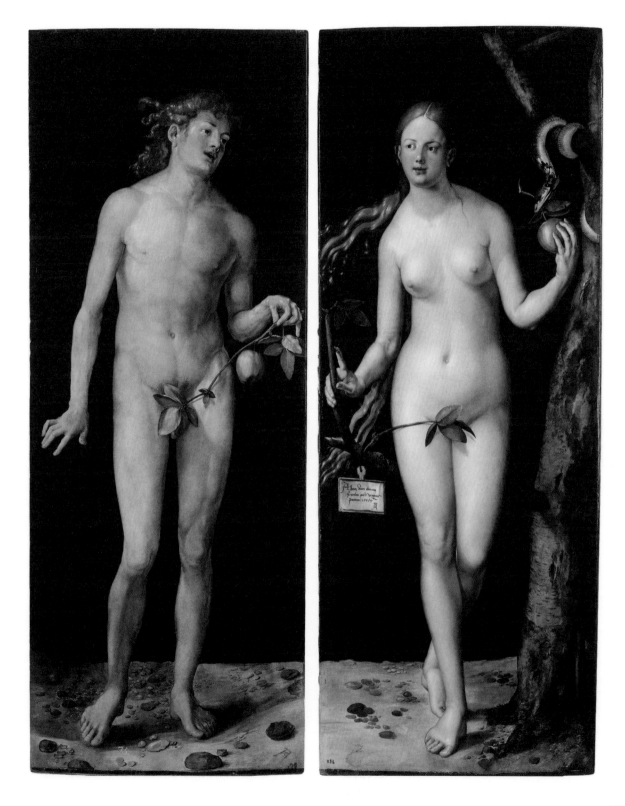

Four Books on Human Proportion (1528)

Pages from Dürer's *Four Books on Human Proportion* show his desire to depict the human anatomy in all its imperfection, not purely as an idealised model. Above left: A slightly overweight man. Above right: A young boy. Below left: An unconventional male pose, indicating muscle groups. Below right: An older woman leaning on a cane.

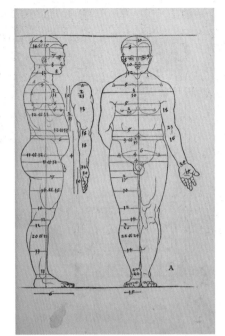

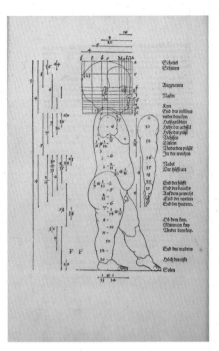

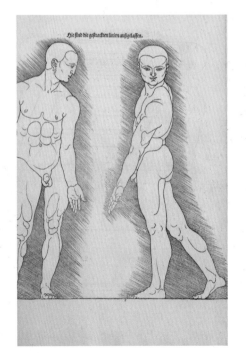

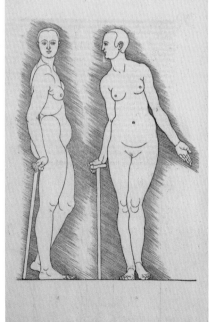

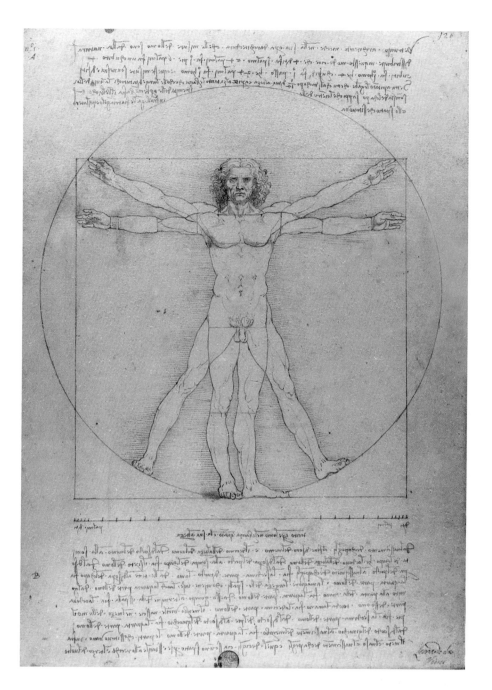

Leonardo da Vinci

Vitruvian Man (1490). Da Vinci's version of the ideal human figure, as defined by the Roman architect Vitruvius in the first century BCE.

is Albrecht Dürer's first book, written by himself. This book I improved and handed to the printer in 1528. Albrecht Dürer.'

It was a book of anatomy for artists, not anatomists. More than that, it offered a radical view of the body which departed from the accepted standard of the ideal man and woman. That standard had been laid down by a Roman architect, Vitruvius, in the first century BCE. Vitruvius' great work, *De architectura* (*On Architecture*) describes the perfect proportions for buildings of various kinds; but it digresses long enough to prescribe the ideal proportions of the human body, from which – he argued – all ideal proportions derived.

The navel is naturally placed in the centre of the human body, and, if in a man lying with his face upward, and his hands and feet extended, from his navel as the centre, a circle be described, it will touch his fingers and toes. It is not alone by a circle, that the human body is thus circumscribed, as may be seen by placing it within a square. For measuring from the feet to the crown of the head, and then across the arms fully extended, we find the latter measure equal to the former; so that lines at right angles to each other, enclosing the figure, will form a square.

Vitruvius was long forgotten when a copy of *De architectura* resurfaced in the library of the monastery at St Gallen in Switzerland in 1414. It fed the Renaissance hunger for the classical world and Leon Battista Alberti drew heavily on it for his own book *De re aedificatoria* (*On the Subject of Buildings*) in 1450. Artists aspired to illustrate the Vitruvian man, most famously Leonardo da Vinci in 1490.

The Vitruvian man was a theoretical version of perfection; but no human body is perfect. Dürer's innovation was to acknowledge that imperfection with a set of images for over a dozen different body types. Each image showed the size of parts of the body as fractions of the whole. He acknowledged Vitruvius, and was clearly influenced by Alberti and da Vinci; but his studies of ordinary bodies, real bodies, were a deviation from tradition. They were based, as he noted, on 'two to three hundred living persons' (not long-dead ideals). 'I hold,' he wrote, 'that the perfection of form and beauty is contained in the sum of all men.' And not, he might have added, in any one human being. It was an egalitarian approach.

The first two books of the quartet contain Dürer's examples – thirteen of them. The third explains how the proportions can be further modified to give a more or less infinite variety of realistic body shapes. His techniques include mathematical ways of distorting shape in the manner of a concave or convex mirror. The fourth book considers how anatomy regulates movement, and therefore what makes for a convincing pose in a painted scene. It also contains an essay in which Dürer agonises over what constitutes beauty: an ideal or a reality. Although *Human Proportion* is not a textbook of dissection, it illustrates well the broader appeal of anatomy in the sixteenth century, part of a move away from 'perfection' to reality, an imitation of nature as it actually appeared.

6 Michelangelo

Florence was the epicentre of the Renaissance and Michelangelo (1475–1564), who grew up surrounded by its manifestations, was a prodigious talent even as a child. At the age of fourteen he was apprenticed to the artist Domenico Ghirlandaio, whose team were engaged in decorating the Sistine Chapel. In his own work, Ghirlandaio painted scenes of everyday life, and even his religious compositions were humanised by the inclusion of ordinary people and patrons. He was so impressed by Michelangelo that he began to pay him when he was only fourteen, and recommended him as one of his two best students to Lorenzo de' Medici, Lorenzo the Magnificent, that great patron of the Renaissance arts.

If there is no evidence for Dürer having practised dissection, there is plenty for Michelangelo. As a young man he attended at least one public dissection. It so fascinated him that he asked the Santo Spirito convent in Florence for permission to dissect cadavers from its hospital awaiting burial. In return, Michelangelo presented the convent with an anatomically accurate crucifix of a naked Christ, nearly 1.5m (5ft) in height, in 1492, when he was just seventeen.

His grasp of the subject was, according to his contemporaries, unequalled; and in his vast output, his convincing depictions of the human form demand the viewer's attention. They are recognisable, familiar in face and action, not mere memes in conventional poses, but real people conveying emotion and exhibiting tension in muscle and sinew.

Michelangelo's people are famous: God and Man in his depiction of the Creation on the roof of the Sistine Chapel (1512); the statue of David (1504), the biblical hero who killed the giant Goliath, on which even the blood vessels on the back of David's powerful hands are visible. He was a master of painting, but a genius of sculpture. One of his earliest works is the *Battle of the Centaurs* (1492), a low-relief scene of hand-to-hand combat reminiscent of Antonio del Pollaiuolo's *Battle of the Nude Men*, but a tour de force of three-dimensional visualisation and dexterity.

In contrast to the virility of David and the explosive moment of God's creation of Man, two early depictions of the Virgin Mary positively glow with gentle motherhood. His *Pietà* (1499), now in St Peter's Basilica in the Vatican, depicts Mary's grief as she cradles her dead son. The limp body sags, all tension gone from its muscles. His *Madonna and Child* (1504) was also his first work to leave Italy, bought by two wealthy Italian cloth merchants in Bruges. It captures the pride and serenity of a mother, more than the holiness of the Virgin, and breaks with tradition in its grouping. Europe is full of standard Madonna and Child portrayals: Mary, in blue, with a halo, staring out at the viewer, indicating peace with two fingers of her right hand and cradling the often strangely mature baby Jesus in her left arm. The Bruges Madonna is herself at peace, right arm completely relaxed, left arm steadying but not restraining the toddler Christ, who seems to be about to set off out into the world to begin his mission. Her work is done. Albrecht Dürer saw Michelangelo's *Madonna and Child* during his travels as a woodcutter journeyman.

At the other end of his life, Michelangelo was commissioned to paint *The Last Judgement* (1541) on a wall of the Sistine Chapel. The immense scene, in which the world ends and all men are judged by God to be fit for either heaven or hell, gave Michelangelo

In 1504, Michelangelo's statue, which portrays the boy who slew the giant Goliath, evoked the defence of civil liberties in the threatened city state of Florence. Its eyes are directed defiantly toward Rome. Today it is a symbol of perfect youth and vigour.

infinite scope for portrayals of human bodies in a range of positions and emotions as they rise from the dead. At the centre sits Jesus in judgement – not the bearded victim of crucifixion, but a clean-shaven, powerful young man. And at Jesus' left foot sits a man holding a scalpel in one hand and his own flayed skin in the other. The figure is St Bartholomew, who was martyred by being flayed alive, but the skin he holds up bears the face of Michelangelo. If there were any doubt about Michelangelo's enthusiasm for anatomy, this removes it.

He returned to dissection frequently during his life, and in old age began a project with Paduan anatomist Realdo Colombo (1516–59). Colombo had trained at the Universities of Padua and Pisa and was Michelangelo's physician in Rome while the artist was designing the dome of St Peter's. Michelangelo was to provide the illustrations for Colombo's anatomical text. The project was never realised, either because of Michelangelo's advanced age or because of Colombo's early death aged only forty-four. It's a tantalising prospect. What we now regard as the most important book in the history of modern anatomy had been published in 1543 (Vasalius's *De humani corporis fabrica*) only five years before Colombo's arrival in Rome. Could his partnership with Michelangelo have produced something even better?

7 Realdo Colombo

Colombo's text was eventually printed by his son after his death in 1559. *De re anatomica libri XV (Fifteen Books about Anatomy)* shines a light on his working practices. He was evangelical about practical anatomy, including animal vivisection, as the only way of discovering for oneself how the body worked. The title page is a graphic image of a public dissection. Everyone in attendance, including an artist, is playing close attention, except for one old man with his head buried in a book. Colombo was critical of Galen, and of anyone who unquestioningly repeated Galen's errors. Much of his antagonism stemmed from Galen's assumptions about human anatomy being based largely on that of animals, although as far as is known Colombo too only conducted vivisection on animals. Colombo, however, had far more experience of human cadavers than Galen ever had.

De re anatomica takes an innovative approach to its subject. Instead of considering each organ individually and separately discussing the nerves and blood supply, Colombo wrote about each organ and the vessels that supply it – which are, after all, integral to its function. It was a radical perspective and, with it, Colombo was able to discover the pulmonary circuit, a vital step between Da Vinci's recognition of the heart as a pump and William Harvey's discovery of circulation. Individual books within *De re anatomica* are devoted to various organs, to the skeleton, to muscles, to ligaments and cartilage, to glands and to the skin. Book Fourteen is devoted to

BELOW
Madonna della Pietà (1498–9)

A sculptural meeting of naturalism and Renaissance idealism, Michelangelo's *Pietà* is the only work he ever signed. It embodies the stillness of grief.

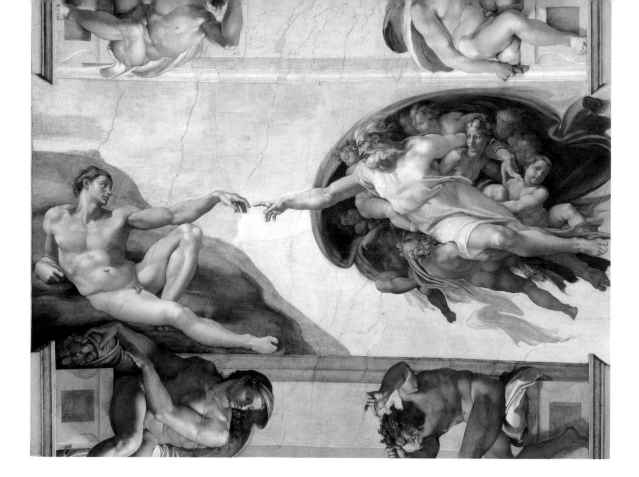

the value of vivisection; and Book Fifteen, delightfully, contains a list from Colombo's personal experiences of 'things rarely seen in anatomy'.

Colombo is credited with naming the placenta and correctly identifying its function. And although he was not the first to discover the clitoris, he was the first to identify it as a primarily sexual organ. The news came as a shock to some Renaissance men who feared that, if women had a sexual organ, an authentic appendage, they might be anatomically the equal of men, or – worse still – have the potential to be hermaphroditic, rendering men redundant.

8 Andreas Vesalius

Realdo Colombo's *De re anatomica* is often overlooked in favour of the book which appeared just before his arrival in Rome, *De humani corporis fabrica libri septem* (*On the Fabric of the Human Body in Seven Books*) by Andreas Vesalius. Today regarded as the most influential book of anatomy ever published, it was in its time not without detractors – among them, Realdo Colombo.

The two men were acquainted, and Colombo covered for Vesalius at the University of Padua while the latter oversaw the production of his book in Basel in 1543. Vesalius credited Colombo, his 'very good friend', with many of the discoveries in *De humani*

God giving life to man, on the ceiling of the Sistine Chapel in the Vatican. The chapel is named after Pope Sixtus IV who commissioned the finest artists of the day to paint its frescoes.

De humani corporis
fabrica (1543)

The frontispiece of Vesalius'
landmark work depicts a
wooden anatomy theatre
standing within a larger
pillared hall. A skeleton
among the crowd oversees the
dissection of the abdomen of
a woman, while dogs and a
monkey wait for scraps of offal.

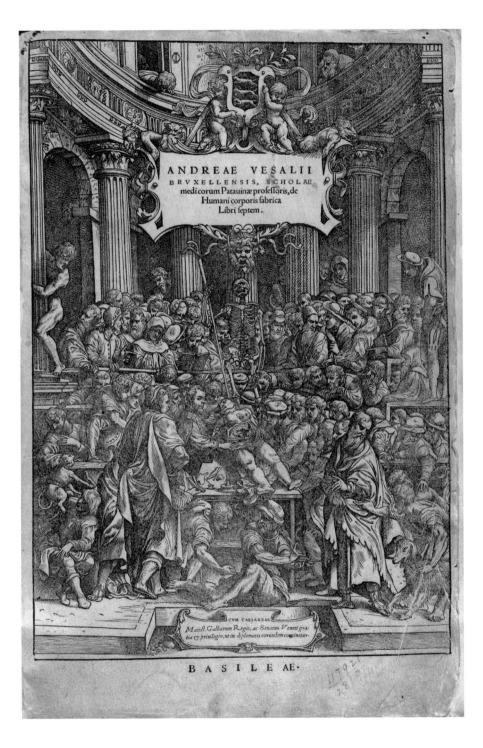

ANDREAE VESALII
BRVXELLENSIS, SCHOLAE
medicorum Patauinæ profeſſoris, de
Humani corporis fabrica
Libri ſeptem.

CVM CAESAREAE
Maieſt. Galliarum Regis, ac Senatus Veneti gra-
tia & priuilegio, ut in diplomatis eorundem continetur.

BASILEAE.

corporis fabrica. However, Colombo undermined Vesalius at Padua by pointing out mistakes in his teaching to Vesalius's students. Colombo's central complaint was that Vesalius, despite being a critic of Galen, was making the same mistakes as Galen by basing his work on the anatomy of animals. For example, he used animal bones to illustrate lectures on the human skeleton, thereby implicitly supporting Galen. One of Vesalius's errors was to assume details of the human eye based on that of a cow. Although both men were proponents of animal vivisection in the interests of the science, Colombo was the only one to take advantage of it. They fell out. By 1555 Vesalius was calling his former colleague an ignoramus and claiming to have taught him everything he knew. It was neither the first nor the last academic spat.

Vesalius (1514–64) was born Andries van Wesel in Brussels but is better known by the Latin form of his name. He came from a medical family: his great grandfather graduated from the University of Pavia and taught medicine at the University of Leuven, where Vesalius himself studied; his grandfather was the personal physician to Holy Roman Emperor Maximilian I; and his father was Maximilian's apothecary. For a while, Vesalius studied Galen in Paris, digging up bones in the Cemetery of the Innocents to get greater insight. His PhD in Leuven was on the writings of that early critic of Galen, Rhazes.

De humani corporis fabrica explicitly set out to advance anatomy beyond Galen. Even before its publication, Vesalius's contradiction of Galen was controversial. Galen had been accepted as accurate for centuries; and the fact that he based his observations on the organs and vessels of animals had been forgotten. It was Vesalius's rediscovery of this fact that prompted him to write *De humani corporis fabrica*.

His challenge to the received wisdom of Galen met with resistance and accusations of disrespect. He had to temper his criticism, for example, by acknowledging that Galen was correct, but not about humans. Vesalius was especially strong on the skeleton: he was the first to correctly describe the elements of the sternum, the sacrum and the sphenoid and temporal bones of the skull. His book refuted over 300 of Galen's errors, including one easy to disprove, that the human lower jawbone was in two parts like those of other animals. Vesalius also corrected the Galenic belief that men have fewer ribs than women – because of the so-called spare rib taken from the first man from which God created the first woman. This had repercussions for anatomy's relationship with the Christian Church, for whom the spare rib story was central to its origin myth and to the Church's belief that men were superior to women.

He confirmed, as Berengario had done, the absence of the rete mirabile in human anatomy. He disproved Galen's theory that blood originated in the liver, and that it passed through micropores from the left ventricle of the heart to the right – one of many instances in which Vesalius's first-hand observation through dissection contradicted Galen's teaching. Vesalius gave by far the best anatomy of the brain to date. He presented new details about the digestive system and the blood vessels, although in the latter case he was still unable to counter the Galenic principle that the veins and arteries were two separate blood systems.

One glaring error by Vesalius was to repeat Galen's view of the female organs of reproduction, which the Greek physician based on those of a dog he had dissected. It's to Vesalius's credit that he corrected the error for the second edition of *De humani corporis*

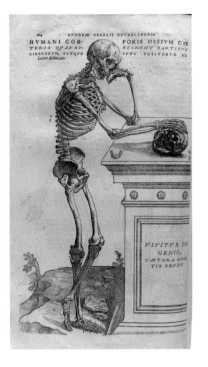

De humani corporis fabrica (1543)

Vesalius' illustrations were drawn by Jan Stephans van Calcar, a Dutchman working in Italy. Above: A skeleton, legs crossed, ponders the future. The skull which it holds sits on a tomb on which is inscribed, in Latin, 'Genius lives on; all else is mortal.' Right: A flayed body, suspended by a rope through its eye sockets from a wall, displays the muscles of the limbs and the cavity behind the ribcage. Opposite: A front view of a flayed body shows the muscles of the neck, shoulders, limbs and abdomen, set against an Italian landscape.

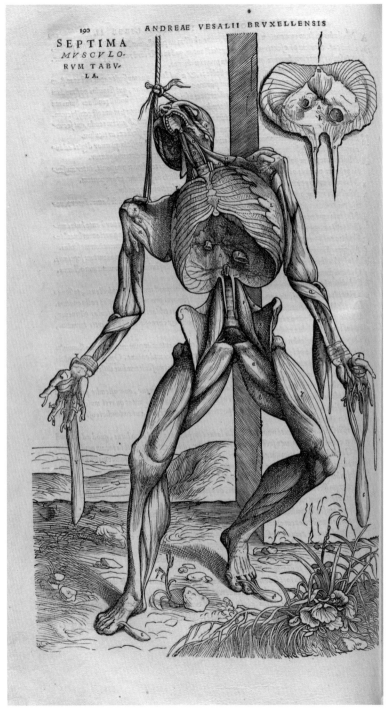

PRIMA MVSCV-
LORVM TABVLA.

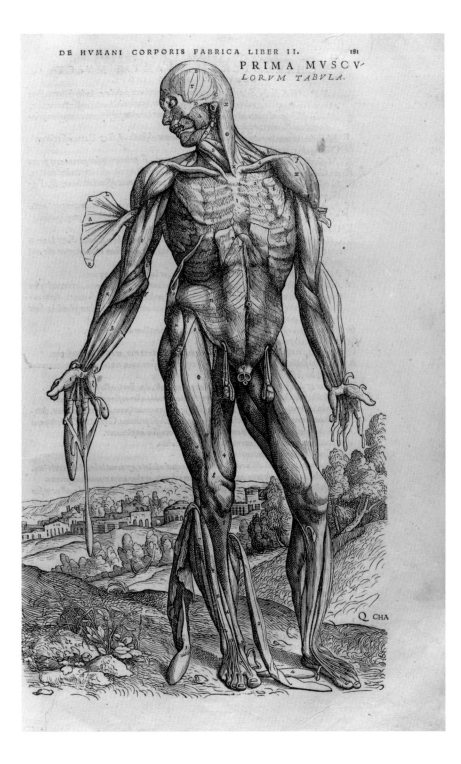

Q CHA

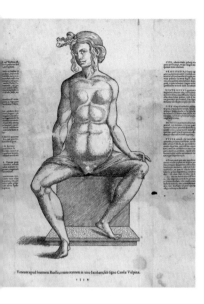

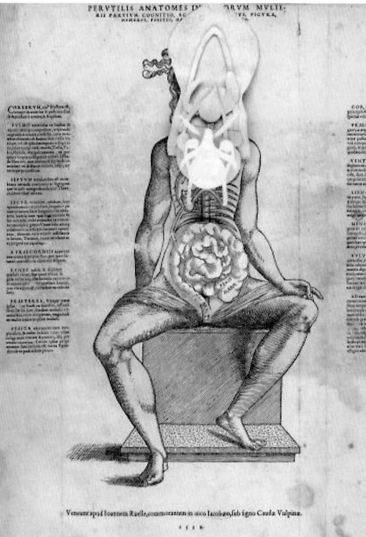

Fugitive sheet of female anatomy (1538)

Heinrich Vogtherr pioneered the use of pressed linen flaps to recreate the process of dissection by revealing different layers of anatomy. This example has four levels: the exterior (above); the organs and digestive system (right); the reproductive system; and the skeleton.

fabrica in 1555, replacing the original image of the placenta and foetal membrane with a more accurate one. He retained his curiosity about anatomy to the end of his life; Vesalius was preparing a third edition when he died, after being shipwrecked on the island of Zakynthos, aged forty-nine.

The illustrations in the seven books of *De humani corporis fabrica* are rich in realistic detail. They are almost certainly drawn from life, as it were, by an artist present at a dissection; and they reflect all the advances in human representation and in printing techniques which the Renaissance brought. They are very fine woodcuts, and the original artwork may have been executed by Jan Stephan van Calcar, a pupil of the great Venetian artist Titian. Bodies are drawn as if they were classical Greek sculptures, posed artfully and with limbs ending at the shoulder or thigh like a statue, if not required for the subject of the illustration. They are elegant and informative.

Best of all, they have flaps, so that in imitation of the process of dissection, the reader can lift an organ out of the way to find out what lies behind it. This was not the first use of such a device: in 1538 Heinrich Vogtherr (1490–1556), an artist with his own printworks in Strasbourg, produced an anatomy with fugitive sheets (the technical name for a flap which flies away to reveal hidden details). Although his book design was innovative, Vogtherr's anatomy was not. In one illustration he includes the lacmamil, a pair of non-existent ducts leading to the nipples which were thought to transform blood into breast milk. The French physician Jean Ruel (1474–1537), published a series of fugitive sheets in 1539, with which the viewer could peel away the layers of male and female anatomy. Ruel is also notable for a compilation of all the veterinary knowledge of ancient Greece and Rome, *Hippiatrika* or *Veterinariae medicinae* (1530). *Veterinariae medicinae* (*Veterinary Medicine*) is of interest to all bibliophiles because it includes an early contents page and glossary.

Vesalius's *De humani corporis fabrica* presented in every sense the state of the art and science of anatomy to its readers. It made significant breaks with the past, not only in revealing Galen's feet of clay but by being purely and scientifically anatomical. Even Mondino and Berengario, modernists in many ways, had felt obliged to include elements of Galenic philosophy in their discussions. Vesalius was only interested in scientific truth.

It was an instant bestseller, and an abridged version *De humani corporis fabrica librorum epitome* (*Abridgement of On the Fabric of the Human Body*), published at around the same time with an eye on the student market, sold even better – that version included a cut-out-and-keep page of anatomical details from which students could construct their own fugitive sheets. More than 700 copies of the first two editions of *De humani corporis fabrica* survive, including a unique hand-coloured version bound in imperial purple. Vesalius presented this special edition to the Holy Roman Emperor Charles V, to whom he

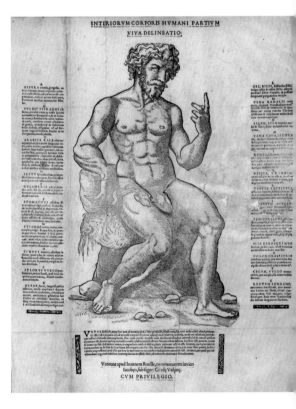

had dedicated the book. Soon after its publication Charles hired Vesalius as imperial physician, the same role his grandfather had played for Charles's father Maximilian. One copy currently held by Brown University in the United States was – aptly but gruesomely – rebound in a cover of human skin for the Paris International Exposition in 1867 by Vesalius's fellow Bruxellois, the bookbinder Josse Schavye. There is no record of the original owner of either the book or the skin.

The popularity of Vesalius's book also helped to popularise the use of flaps. Only a year after its publication, Jacob Frölich of Strasbourg published two fugitive sheets with the title *Anathomia oder abconterfettung eynes Mans leib, wie er inwendig gestaltet ist* (*Anatomy, or Depiction of the human body as it appears internally*). The images of a man, with six flaps, and a woman, with nine, were surrounded by three columns of German text and numerous smaller woodcuts of individual organs in greater detail.

9 Charles Estienne

Vesalius was the victim of counterfeiters, including the Flemish copperplate artist Thomas Lambrit, who copied Vesalius's illustrations, and Gyles Godet, a French publisher working in London who copied Lambrit's. A fellow student of Vesalius, Charles Estienne, was the object of several accusations of plagiarism, both during his lifetime and after it.

Estienne (1504–64) and Vesalius were classmates in Paris. Their tutor, Jacques

De dissectione partium corporis humani (1545)

Right: On a page from Charles Estienne's anatomy a male figure hangs his skull cap on a tree and bends forward to reveal the contents of the skull. Far right: A pregnant female figure in palatial surroundings displays her reproductive system. Opposite: Publication of Charles Estienne's book was delayed by accusations of the plagiarism of its images, including this detailed diagram of the skeleton.

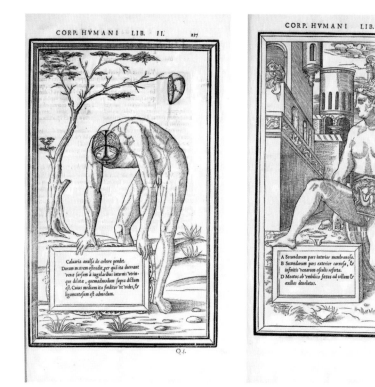

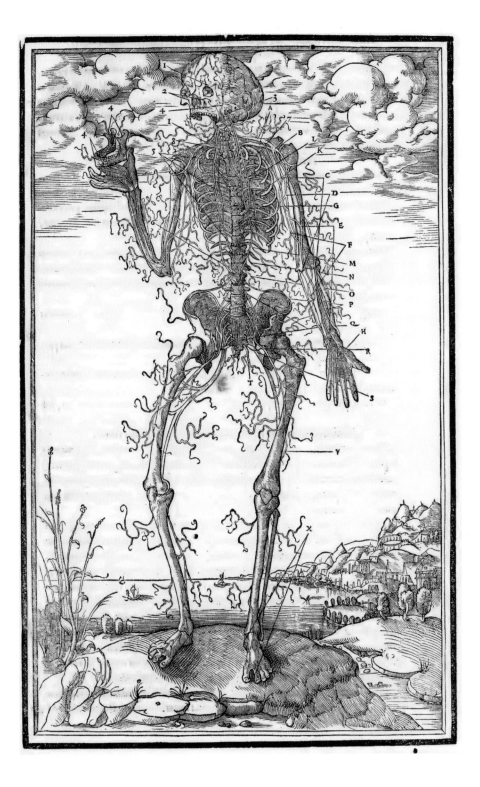

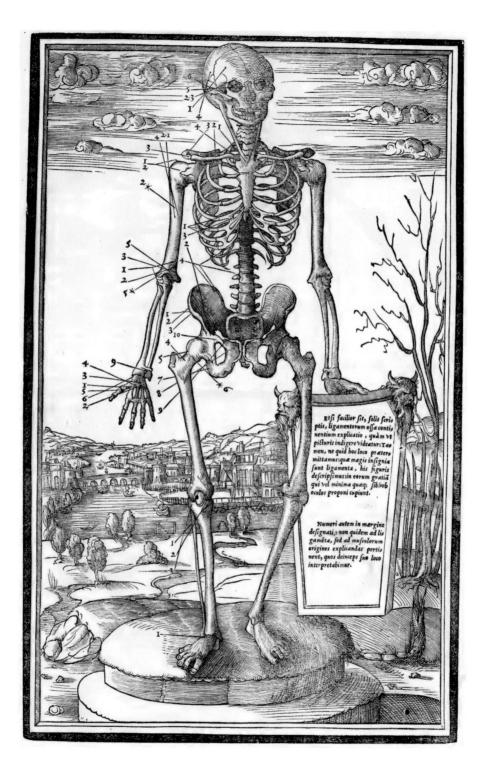

Etsi facilior sit, solis scrip
tis, ligamentorum ossa conti
nentium explicatio, quàm ut
picturis indigere videatur: Ta
men, ne quid hoc loco præter
mittamus:quæ magis insignia
sunt ligamenta, his figuris
descripsimus:in eorum gratiã
qui vel minima quæq; sub ob
oculos proponi cupiunt.

Numeri autem in margine
designati, non quidem ad lis
gaméta, sed ad musculorum
origines explicandas pertio
nent, quos deinceps suo loco
interpretabimur.

Dubois, taught exclusively through animal dissection, and relied on Berengario's text; so, it's no coincidence that both gifted students saw the need for a better anatomy. Estienne was quickest to address the shortcoming, with the text and illustrations of his *De dissectione partium corporis humani libri tres* (*On the Dissection of the Parts of the Human Body, in Three Books*) ready for publication in 1539, four years ahead of Vesalius.

Production was halted, however, by a lawsuit from another classmate of Estienne's. Étienne de Rivière had asked Estienne to translate his own work from French into Latin, and now accused him of plagiarising it. The case was resolved when Estienne agreed to credit de Rivière for details and illustrations of the dissection process. Publication of *De dissectione* was delayed by the dispute until 1545 and to Vesalius went the glory.

Had *De dissectione* been printed in 1539, as planned, it would certainly have stolen some of Vesalius's thunder. It contained some pioneering observations, and its model of the brain was bettered only by Vesalius's. However, de la Rivière's text may not have been the only element that Estienne stole. His images are a very mixed bunch, of variable quality and style. Some, of figures in clearly erotic poses, seem to have been copied from a set of fifteen pornographic prints called *The Loves of the Gods*, engraved in 1527 by Jacopo Caraglio. In these cases, the most explicit parts of the image have been cut out of the print block for Estienne's book, and internal anatomy literally inserted into the gap; it's possible to see the joins between the inserted block and its erotic surroundings. It's not clear why Estienne chose this approach, but perhaps the lawsuit, and Vesalius's success, constrained his woodcut budget. The images certainly devalue the undoubted quality of the text.

10 Conrad Gessner

It's noticeable that as human anatomy at last began to distance itself from the errors of animal dissection, books of zoology began to appear in their own right. Animal medicine has been practiced since at least 3000 BCE. An Egyptian papyrus is the oldest known veterinary book, written in around 1900 BCE. But as Jean Ruel demonstrated in his *Veterinariae medicinae*, much has been written since then. The first modern veterinary book, inasmuch as it was published soon after Vesalius, was written by Conrad Gessner (1516–65) of Zurich, who was the city's chief (human) physician. His *Historia animalium* (*History of Animals*), published in volumes between 1551 and 1558 was the first book in which animals were depicted realistically and in their natural habitats.

Historia animalium borrowed its title from an earlier book by Aristotle but took a more scientific approach to describing the natural history of the world. It was generously illustrated and became by far the most successful book of its type during the Renaissance. Medieval bestiaries had long been popular sources of entertainment, although they often contained wildly inaccurate portrayals of animals, both real and fantastical. Gessner, ever the scientist, included imaginary beasts, but identified them as such – sometimes to the disappointment of his publishers, who unscrupulously inserted further sensational, mythological animals to spice up the book. Although not a pure anatomy, *Historia animalium* contains coloured images and notes about each animal's attributes, habits, occurrence in the arts and use in medicine and diet.

Gessner's lead illustrator was Lucas Schan, an ornithologist from Strasbourg. Many artists contributed, and Gessner was not above 'borrowing' the work of others. The book

De dissectione partium corporis humani (1545)

A skeletal anatomy with details of the joints of the arms and legs.

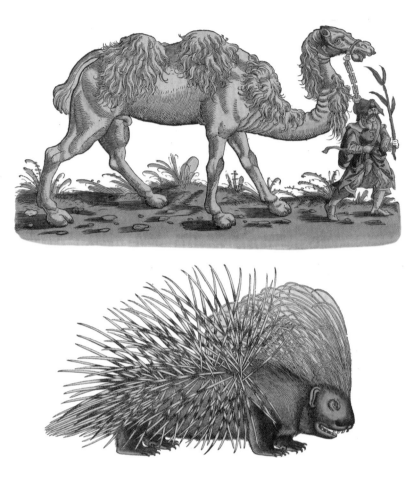

Historiae animalium (1551)

Top: The camel in Conrad Gessner's bestiary shows an awareness of anatomy in the musculature of the animal's legs. Bottom: Gessner concurred with the popular belief that the porcupine could fire its quills like arrows at any predator.

includes Albrecht Dürer's famous picture of a rhinoceros, an animal which neither Gessner nor Dürer had ever seen. Gessner was, however, well travelled and made notes of local wildlife wherever he went throughout his life, epitomising the new Renaissance style of observational science. The pictures were so popular that a second book was published, *Icones animalium* (*Pictures of Animals*). *Historia animalium* has the rare distinction among zoological works of being placed on the Catholic Church's list of banned books – not because of any heresy of natural history but because Conrad Gessner was a Protestant.

11 Juan Valverde de Amusco

Andreas Vesalius's *De humani corporis fabrica* was sensational not only for anatomy but for the publishing industry. Counterfeiters and imitators rushed to cut themselves a slice of the book's success. Vesalius was greatly irritated by these hangers-on. Other writers, following in his wake, did so precisely because of the contribution he had made to the science. By popularising it he drew other physicians into it, some of whom were able to build on his great foundations.

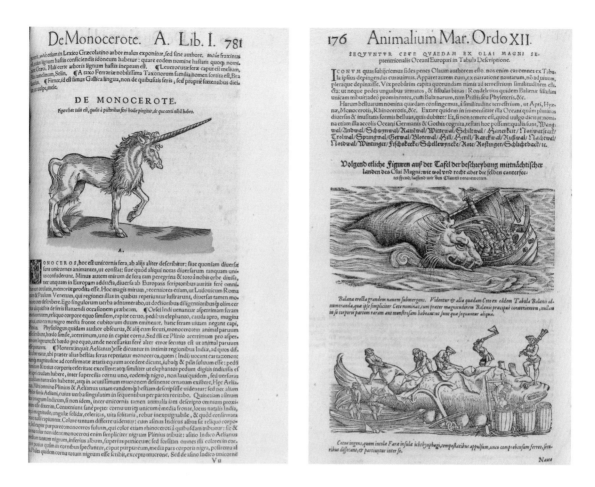

The Latin text within the images reads as follows:

De Monocerote. A. Lib. I. 781

DE MONOCEROTE.

Figu hæc talis eft, qualis à pictoribus fieri hodie pingitur, de qua certi nihil habeo.

A.

176 Animalium Mar. Ordo XII.

Volgend etliche Figuren auß der Tafel der beschreybung mittnächtischer landen des Olai Magni: wie wol vnd recht aber die selben conterfeetet syend/lassend wir den Olaum verantworten.

Nauta

Juan Valverde de Amusco (1525–*c*.1589) was a rare Spanish entry into the arena. He published several books on anatomy, including *De animi et corporis sanitate tuenda libellus* (*A Pamphlet on the Preservation of Mental and Physical Health*) in Paris in 1552 and *Historia de la composicion del cuerpo humano* (*History of the Composition of the Human Body*) in Rome in 1556. His works were printed outside his native Castile, partly because of the greater expertise in image-making in those cities and partly because he himself had studied abroad – at the University of Padua under Realdo Colombo, one of Vesalius's sternest critics.

Perhaps because of his association with Colombo, Vesalius was particularly venomous about Valverde's work, on several grounds. Not only did it carry clear signs of its debt to Colombo; not only was *Historia de la composicion del cuerpo humano* based on his own masterpiece; not only did it dare to make some corrections to Vesalius's work: it had the affrontery to steal its illustrations wholesale from Vesalius's book. Of the forty-two plates in *Historia*, thirty-eight were from *De humani corporis fabrica* and just four were new.

To his credit, Valverde did at least acknowledge his sources. The new plates, however,

ABOVE

Historiae animalium (1551)

Left: Gessner's work, the first modern study of zoology, also included mythical beasts such as the Monocerote, or unicorn. Right: A fantastical sea serpent (above) attacks a ship and a whale (below) is flensed and its organs and oil harvested in barrels.

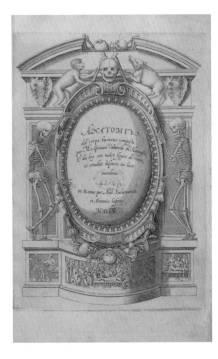

Historia de la composicion del cuerpo humano (1556)

Above: The title page of Juan Valverde's anatomy, which owed a considerable debt to Vesalius. Right: One of the plates which Valverde borrowed from Vesalius' *De humani corporis fabrica*, with its extraordinary view of the head tilted back. Opposite: One of Valverde's original plates, the so-called Muscle Man, in which a male figure holds his skin in one hand, and the flensing knife with which he flayed himself in the other.

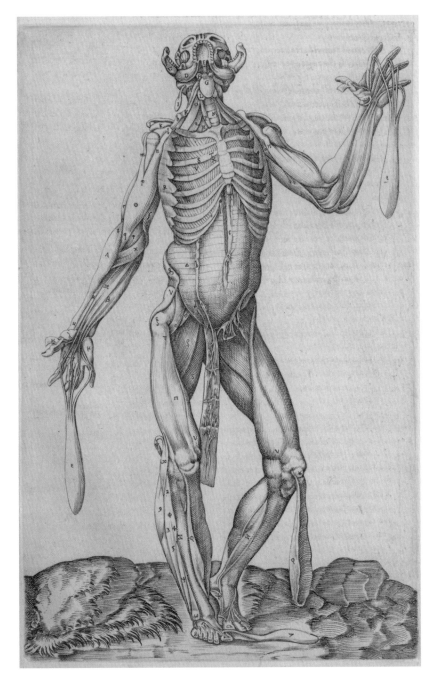

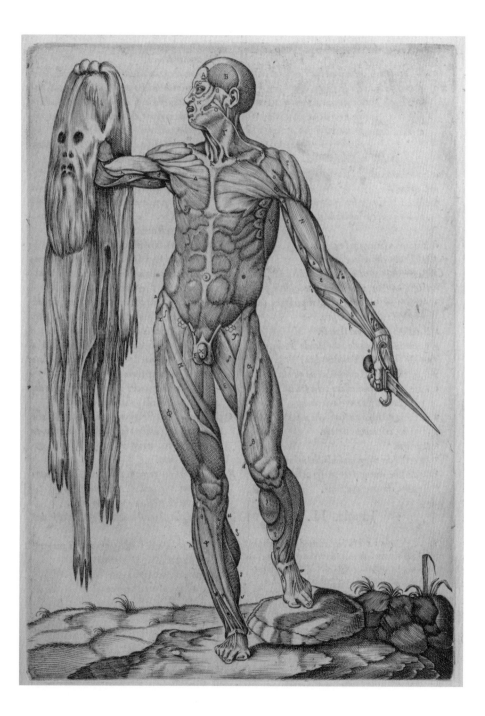

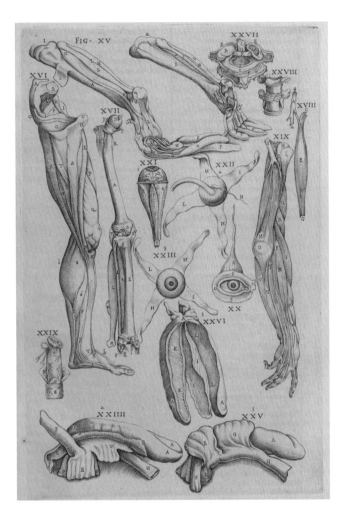

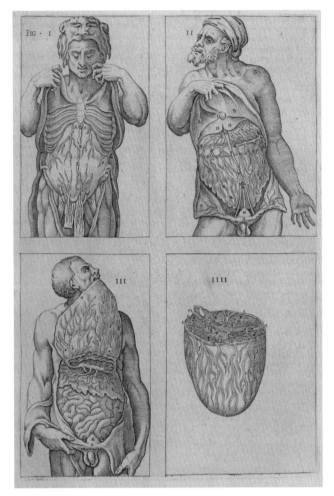

give a fascinating glimpse of what might have emerged from Colombo's proposed collaboration with Michelangelo. Valverde's original artwork was probably by the Spanish artist Gaspar Becerra who had been a pupil of Michelangelo; and the engraver was the Frenchman Nicolas Beatrizet, who had engraved under the direction of Michelangelo between 1540 and 1560. Among the new plates is one known as *Muscle Man*, in which a flayed male figure displays his muscle groups while holding up his own flayed skin in one hand and a flensing knife in the other, an echo of Michelangelo's self-portrait as St Bartholomew in the Sistine's *Last Judgement*. There is much of Michelangelo, and of Colombo, in Valverde's book.

There's no doubt about Valverde's credentials as an anatomist. Although Vesalius attacked him for lacking experience in dissection, that seems unlikely in any student of Colombo. Valverde was particularly interested in the anatomy of the face, and the matters

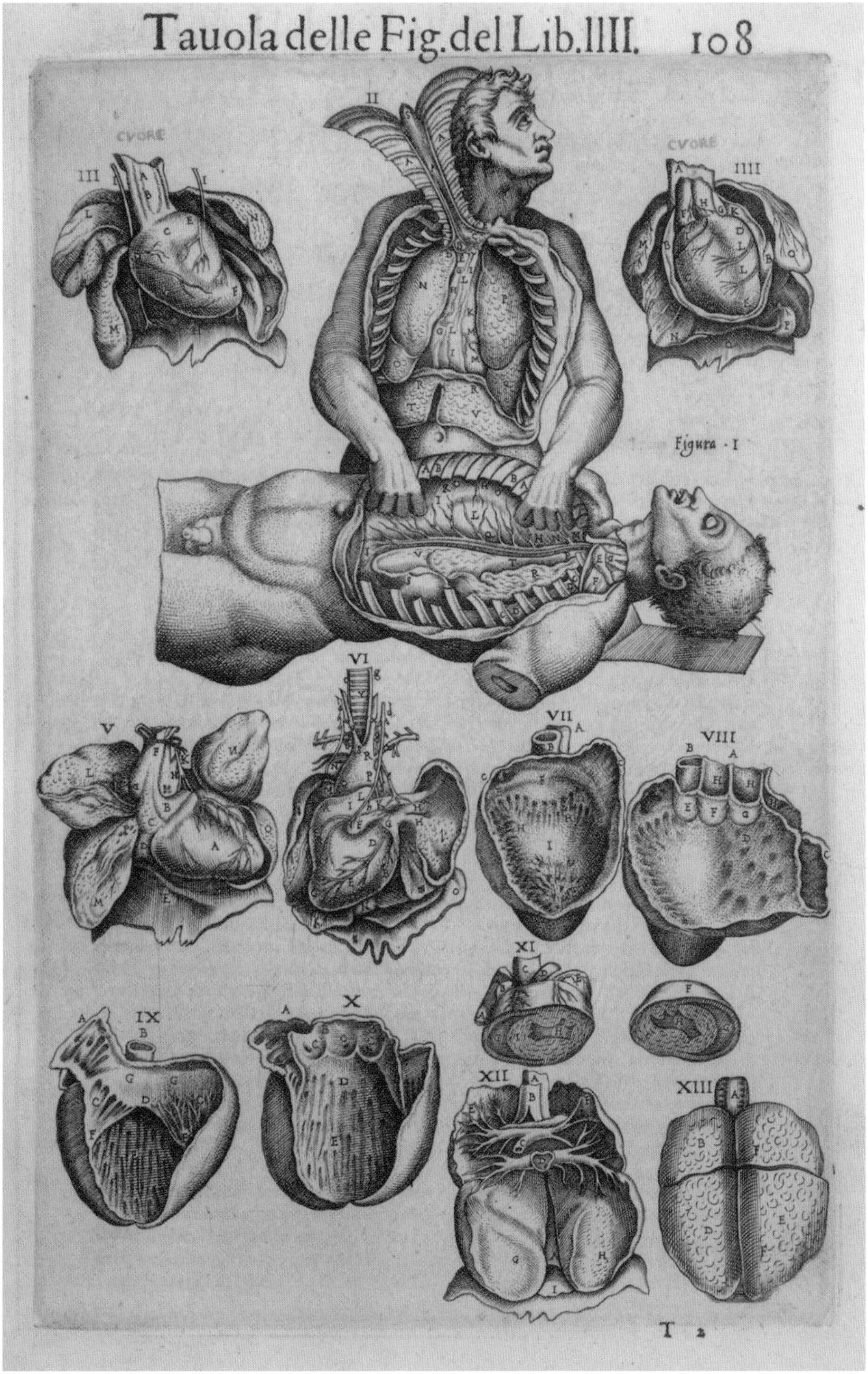

Tauola delle Fig. del Lib. IIII.   108

CVORE

CVORE

Figura · I

T · 2

Historia de la composicion del cuerpo humano (1556)

Juan Valverde reused this plate from Vesalius's *De humani corporis fabrica*, in which one dissected man dissects another, surrounded by details of the heart and lungs.

in which he corrected Vesalius include the muscles of the eyes, nose and larynx. His descriptions of dental anatomy are extremely detailed. Valverde claimed that one reason for writing the book was to improve on Vesalius's rather haphazard organisation of his subject. *Historia de la composicion del cuerpo humano* is one of the more successful imitations of Vesalius and was itself widely read during the sixteenth century.

12 Gabriele Falloppio

If Valverde was Colombo's disciple, then Gabriele Falloppio (1523–62) was Vesalius's successor. Like Vesalius, and Colombo, Falloppio occupied the chair of anatomy at the University of Padua in a short but illustrious career before his early death at the age of thirty-nine. He is remembered today for the Fallopian tube, which connects the ovaries to the uterus, and in describing it he corrected the long-held Galenic belief that the male and female reproductive organs were simply mirrors of each other. One of his main interests was the anatomy of reproduction and sexuality and he conducted what amounts to an early clinical trial in the use of condoms as prophylactics against syphilis. Falloppio reported that of 1,100 soldiers who used a linen sheath, made to measure and soaked in a herbal preparation, none contracted the disease. (Their efficacy in preventing pregnancy was not reported, and only a century later was the use of sheep intestines first recommended for the prevention of both conception and infection.)

Falloppio was an extremely skilled and delicate surgeon, known to have conducted both dissections on cadavers and vivisections on condemned prisoners. His detailed observations led to the discovery of many anatomical elements in the ear – he named the tympanum, the cochlea and the labyrinth. He discovered the Fallopian or facial canal through which the nerves of the face connect with the brain. The Fallopian or pyramidalis muscle in the rectum and the Fallopian or ileocecal valve, which separates the large and small intestines, are also his discoveries. At Padua, the botanical garden, with its supply of medicinal herbs, was also Falloppio's responsibility and today botanists remember him in the genus *Fallopia*, the bindweed family. (Falloppio's name was spelled with two 'p's, but other uses are derived from the Latinised version of his name, with only one.)

He was regarded as an excellent teacher, and the notes of his lectures on several subjects were published after his death. In his lifetime he only published one book, *Gabrielis Falloppii medici mutinensis observationes anatomicae* (*Anatomical Observations of the Modena Physician Gabriele Falloppio*), written as he battled the exhausting tuberculosis which eventually killed him. Published in 1561 – only a year before his death – without illustrations, it not only described his own discoveries but respectfully corrected some of Vesalius's errors. A copy found its way to Vesalius, who overcame his instinctive resistance to criticism and – unaware of Falloppio's passing – wrote him a letter acknowledging Falloppio's eminence. But Vesalius, too, was at the end of his life; the letter was published in May 1564, a month after his own death.

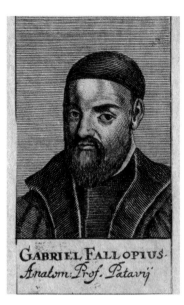

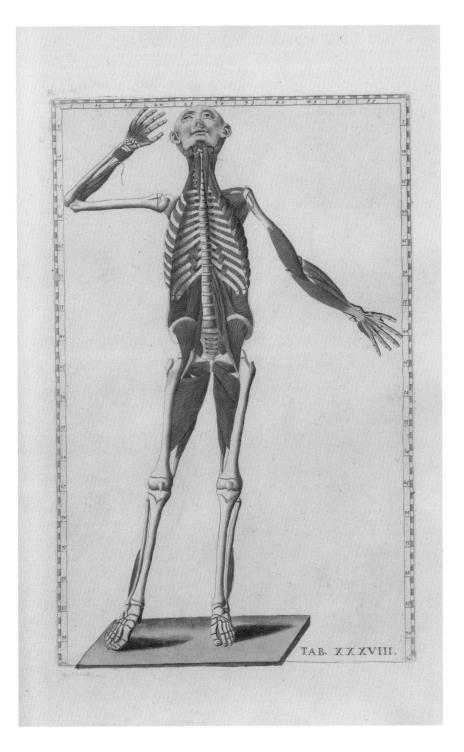

TAB. XXXVIII.

Tabulae anatomicae (1714)

A partially flensed skeleton from Bartolomeo Eustachi's posthumously published work.

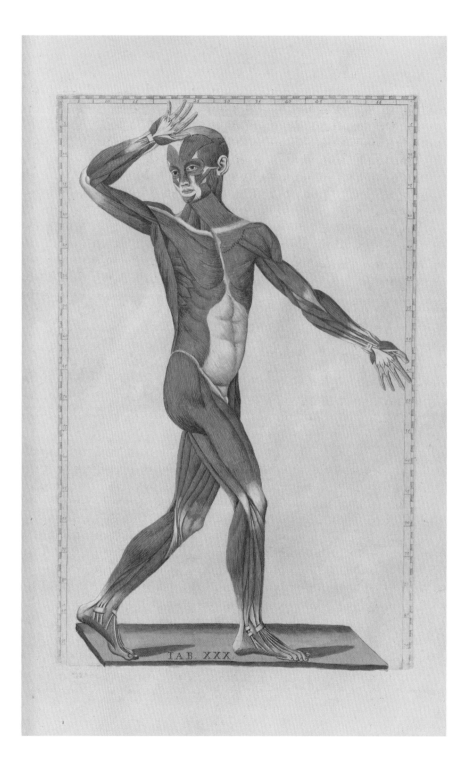

TAB. XXX.

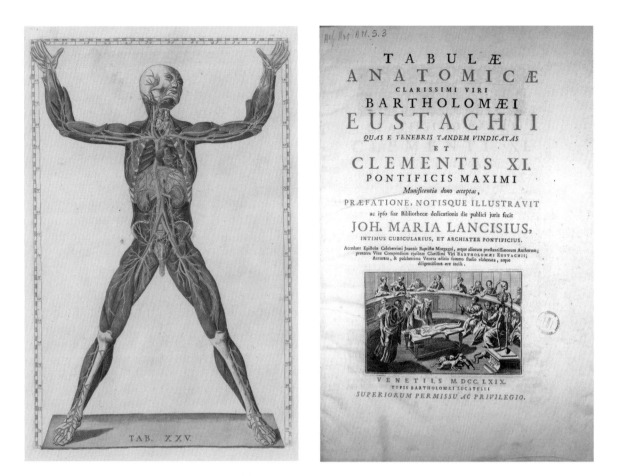

13 Bartolomeo Eustachi

Falloppio was indebted, like all anatomists since, to the groundwork of Vesalius. But for his skills and his improvements on Vesalius's knowledge he may be regarded as the best anatomist of the sixteenth century. Others may have been equally skilled but were somehow overlooked. Bartolomeo Eustachi (c.1500–74), for example, was a fine dissector, a contemporary of Vesalius. He trained at Padua and taught in Rome, and by 1552 he had created forty-seven plates containing the sum of his anatomical knowledge. With Vesalius still in the ascendancy, however, Eustachi could not find a publisher and only eight of his plates were issued as prints in his lifetime. When they were rediscovered in the Vatican library nearly 200 years later by the Italian anatomist Giovanni Maria Lancisi, they revealed a meticulous anatomist making great advances in his subject. The plates were finally published at the expense of Pope Clement XI in 1714, as *Tabulae anatomicae Bartholomaei Eustachii* (*Anatomical Charts of Bartolomeo Eustachi*).

His knowledge of the nervous system was unparalleled in his day, and his exploration of the ear complemented that of Falloppio – the Eustachian tube, part of the middle ear,

Tabulae anatomicae (1714)

Opposite: Muscles of the male anatomy. Above left: Nervous system of the male anatomy. Above right: The title page acknowledges the financial support of Pope Clement XI, who paid for the belated publication of Eustachi's anatomical drawings.

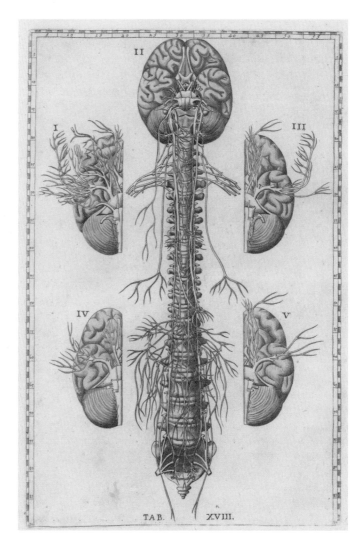

was named in his honour, although the ancient Greek Alcmaeon of Croton was the first to observe it. Eustachi's images are not as artistically styled as those of Vesalius, but they often contain more information. For example, Eustachi's view of the nervous system from the rear depicts a figure standing in a physically awkward position, in order to make more of the system visible to the viewer. The title page of *Tabulae anatomicae* depicts a public anatomy demonstration in which a pack of dogs is shown waiting for discarded organs.

One biographer describes Eustachi as grumpy; perhaps in later life he was bitter about his missed opportunity. Some argue that, had Eustachi been published in his lifetime, he would have been paired with Vesalius as a co-founder of modern anatomy. However, where Vesalius broke with Galen, Eustachi clung to him, a fatal flaw in his position.

14 Ambroise Paré

As the sixteenth century approached its end, a French publication was a reminder that anatomy is essentially a practical science. Ambroise Paré (*c*.1510–90) was a surgeon, specialising in treating the wounds of battle. He served four French kings as royal physician, as good a testament as any to his competence and a remarkable one, since he was unable to heal his first king, Henry II, of a head wound sustained during a jousting tournament in 1559 – a splinter from a lance entered his brain through an eye.

His first book was *La méthode de traicter les playes faites par les arquebuses et aultres bastons à feu* (*The Method of Curing Wounds Caused by Arquebus and Firearms*), printed in Paris in 1545. He published extensively from then on and his collected works (*Les oeuvres d'Ambroise Paré*) were assembled and reprinted in 1575, and translated into Dutch, German and English. Wars were a constant presence for Europeans in the late sixteenth and early seventeenth centuries; the last ten years of Paré's life alone saw the start of wars between England and Spain, between the Dutch and the Portuguese, and between Russia and Sweden, as well as wars of succession for the crowns of Portugal and Poland, a rebellion in Ireland and an internal struggle for control of the Electorate of Cologne. Everyone needed a manual for treating war wounds.

Paré's overriding motive was the alleviation of suffering, and to that end he devised several new surgical techniques. It had, for example, been the practice to cauterise blood vessels during amputation, and to treat them with boiling elder oil. Patients often died, not from amputation, but from the pain and shock of the treatment. Paré was the first surgeon to experiment with ligatures instead of cauterisation, and to treat the wounds with a gentler mixture of rose oil, egg yolk and turpentine. The turpentine acted as an antiseptic, and patients treated with that ointment recovered well. Paré devised several surgical tools, including a primitive ligature called a crow's beak, a forerunner of the haemostatic clamp used today to stop bleeding.

He was interested in neurology and made a study of the phenomenon of phantom pain, which amputees experience after the loss of a limb. Paré deduced that the pain was felt in the brain, not in the stump of the missing limb. His curious mind also investigated the superstitious belief in the use of bezoars (from the Persian for 'antidote'). Bezoars are stones which form in various cavities in the body from indigestible matter from food, hair or plant material. After they were surgically removed from a patient suffering from them, they were prized as objects to be re-swallowed to counter poison. Ox bezoars are still used in Chinese herbal medicine.

Paré found a way of testing the theory. A cook in the French royal court was caught stealing and sentenced to death. Paré persuaded him to take poison as the means, and to ingest a bezoar. The prisoner died in agony seven hours later, proving to Paré's satisfaction that bezoars were not the universal antidotes they were believed to be. (However, modern medicine has found that they can neutralise arsenic.) A plaintiff in an English court in 1603 lost his case when he sued the supplier of an ineffective bezoar; the judgement introduced the legal concept of *caveat emptor* – buyer, beware.

Paré also studied the effects of violent or traumatic death on the organs, and his writings on the subject are considered the beginnings of the science of forensic pathology. His treatise *Reports in Court* offers a structure for recording medical evidence in legal cases.

The Renaissance was an extraordinary time for anatomy, both in art and in science. Its transformation from Galenic theory based on philosophy to evidence-led reality was not completed by the end of the century; elements of Galenism, such as the humors, continued to be accepted in some quarters for another hundred years. But it was the beginning of their end.

Two anatomical milestones marked the end of the sixteenth century. Fittingly, in its final decade, the first purpose-built anatomy theatres were constructed. The University of Padua, which had trained so many of the great sixteenth century anatomists, led the field, in 1594. The University of Leiden followed in 1596, with many more over the following decades. The University of Bologna, where Mondino carried out the first modern dissection in 1315, built its theatre in 1637 – but it constructed it in a building which may first have been used for the purpose in 1563.

One last addition to the anatomist's library appeared in the final years of the century. After the foundational veterinary works of Heinrich Vogtherr and Conrad Gessner, the first thorough anatomy of a non-human species was published in 1598. Carlo Ruini's book *Anatomia del cavallo* (*Anatomy of the Horse*) was published two months after his death, and is a landmark in veterinary literature. Its dramatic illustrations owed much in style to those of Vesalius and were almost as widely plagiarised. Ruini was an admirer of horses. He kept a large stable and rode for pleasure; but despite hailing from Bologna he was not trained either as a physician or an artist and there are errors in his pages. Overall, however, *Anatomia del cavallo* is a symbolic product of its age – an age when warfare and commerce were conducted on horseback, when anatomy was more popular than it had ever been, and when human anatomy was no longer assumed from animal dissections. In Ruini's work, in these unexpected ways, anatomy came of age.

RIGHT

Leiden University anatomy theatre (1596)

A line engraving made soon after the opening of the theatre shows its secondary function as a museum of anatomical exhibits, suspended from the ceiling or – in the form of human and animal skeletons – occupying space within the theatre itself.

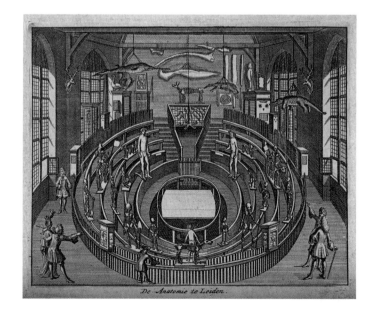

De Anatomie te Leiden.

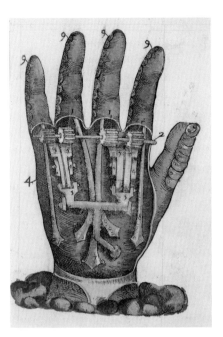

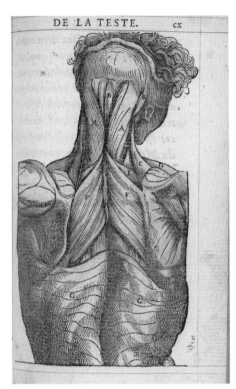

Above: A hand-coloured illustration of the muscles of the back, shoulders and neck. Below: A selection of surgical tools designed by Paré for the treatment of head wounds.

ABOVE

Prosthetic hand (1564)

Ambroise Paré designed several prostheses including hands, limbs, noses and eyes.

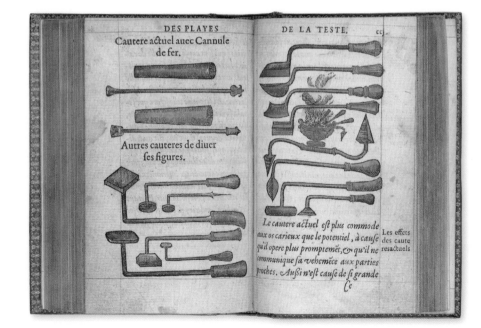

DES PLAYES

Cautere actuel auec Cannule de fer.

Autres cauteres de diuer ses figures.

DE LA TESTE.   cc

Le cautere actuel est plus commode aux os carieux que le potentiel, à cause qu'il opere plus promptemēt, & qu'il ne communique sa vehemēce aux parties proches. Aussi n'est cause de si grande

Les effets des cauteres actuels

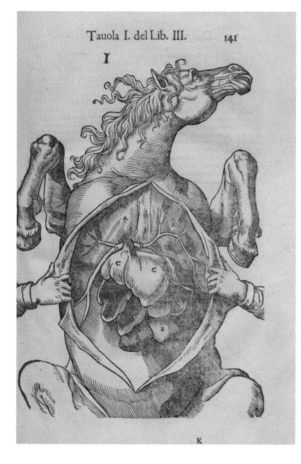

I

K

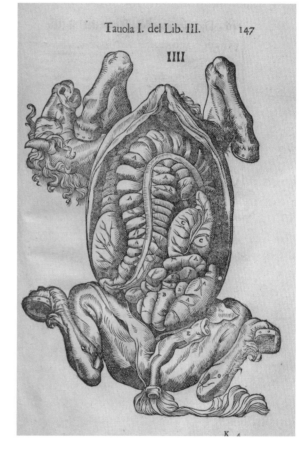

IIII

K 4

Anatomia del cavallo (1598)

Carlo Ruini's book of anatomy was the first
devoted to a non-human species. Above left:
Helping hands reveal the abdominal cavity.
Above right: The male equine anatomy.
Opposite left: The digestive system. Opposite
right: The equine nervous system.

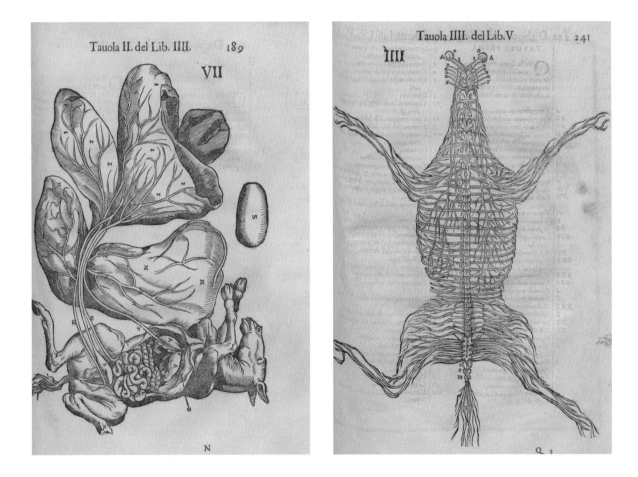

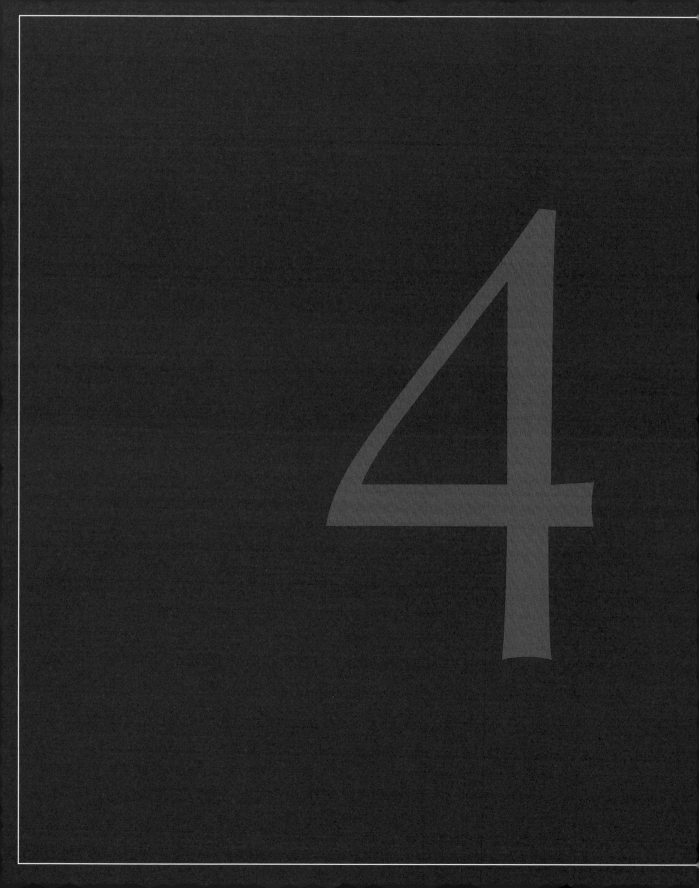

THE AGE OF THE MICROSCOPE
1601–1700

If the sixteenth century was the Big Bang for the modern science of anatomy, the seventeenth century saw the rapid expansion of its universe. The old certainties had been swept away by the flood of the Renaissance, and a new science must be built. As it grew, general anatomists could indulge more in the luxury of specialism and the seventeenth century saw the publication of several works devoted to a single organ. There remained, however, a demand for good general works of anatomy for both the artist and the surgeon.

1 Johann Remmelin

Johann Remmelin made an early contribution to the seventeenth-century shelves of the anatomist's library. His *Catoptrum microcosmicum* (*A Mirror of the Microcosm*) was published in Augsburg in 1613 as a set of fugitive sheets and in 1619 with accompanying text; it ran to several editions during the century. From its original Latin it was translated into French, German, Dutch and English. The choice of languages illustrates the spread of anatomical study northwards through Europe. Padua continued to be the centre of the anatomical world, but in the seventeenth century innovation came from further north, in particular from England.

Remmelin (1583–1632), a native of Ulm in southern Germany, studied medicine in Basel, Switzerland; and it was in 1605, while still a student, that he began to design the plates and flaps of his book. He must have been inspired by earlier books in this form and his own is an ambitious version, with several layers of flaps between the skin and the skeleton. Of the eight copperplates used in the printing, five were devoted to the many levels of anatomy to be revealed in tiny pieces of paper, each one of which must be cut out from the printed sheet and glued in place by hand. It is possible that Remmelin was more excited by the format of the book than by his anatomy classes – *Catoptrum microcosmicum* reflects some ideas that were already out of date by the time of its publication.

Nevertheless, it is a masterpiece of the art of publishing and, errors aside, a useful visual reference for anatomy students and laymen with an interest in the subject. The male torso and the female reproductive system are especially detailed, and the latter – in the first edition – was discreetly covered by a flap depicting the head of a devil. Subsequent editions concealed the anatomy behind a more chaste veil of fabric. The plates were engraved by Lucas Kilian of Augsburg; he learned the skill from his stepfather Dominicus Custos, who worked in the court of Emperor Rudolph II in Prague. Kilian is best known for his engraving of a portrait of Albrecht Dürer, originally painted by Johann Rottenhammer.

Remmelin went on to become the official anatomist for his home town, Ulm. The English-language edition of his book was published in 1675 under the title *A Survey of the*

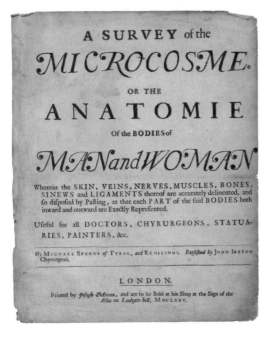

A Survey of the Microcosme or the Anatomie of the Bodies of Man and Woman (1675)

Below: Title page of the English-language edition, printed 'at the sign of the Atlas', of Johann Remmelin's *Catoptrum microcosmicum*. Opposite: One of the fugitive sheets from the English edition of Remmelin's work, carrying the printer Joseph Moxon's dedication to Samuel Pepys on one of the plinths.

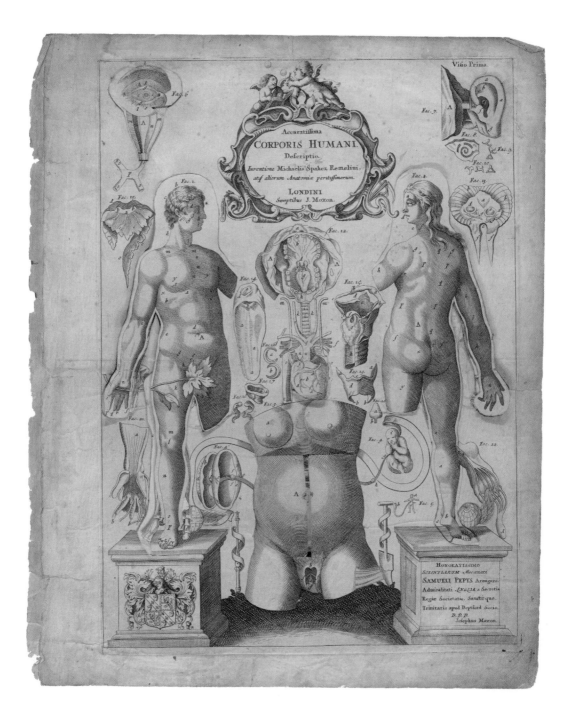

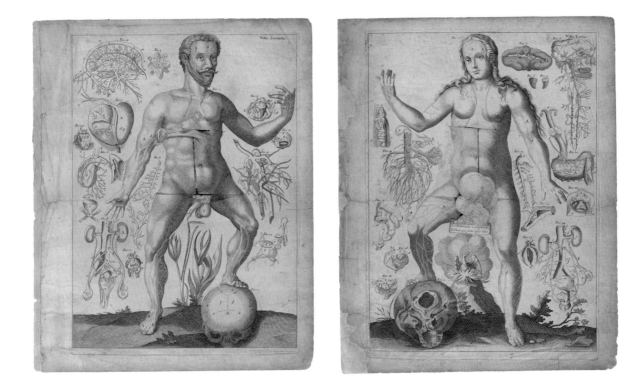

Microcosme, or (to give it its full title) *A Survey of the Microcosme or the Anatomie of the Bodies of Man and Woman wherein the Skin, Veins, Nerves, Muscles, Bones, Sinews and Ligaments Thereof are Accurately Delineated, and so Disposed by Pasting, as that Each Part of the Said Bodies Both Inward and Outward are Exactly Represented. Useful for all Doctors, Chyrurgeons, Statuaries, Painters, Etc.*

The English printer was Joseph Moxon, a fascinating character who learned his craft alongside his father James. Moxon senior printed English Protestant bibles in the Netherlands at a time when the English king was a Catholic. Moxon junior printed Puritan texts during England's republican years, as well as maps and globes – his printshop was to be found 'under the sign of the atlas'. He was a practical man and published several 'how to' guides – on bricklaying, metal and woodworking, printing and, in 1647, *A Book of Drawing, Limning, Washing or Colouring of Mapps and Prints.* He was a keen mathematician, who published paper mathematical instruments and printed the first English-language dictionary of mathematical terms. In 1678 he became the first tradesman to be elected a fellow of the prestigious English scientific institution the Royal Society.

Moxon dedicated his edition of Remmelin to Samuel Pepys in the latter's capacity as Chief Secretary of the Admiralty. The two men knew each other through Moxon's position as the Royal Hydrographer to King Charles II, and Moxon will no doubt have heard Pepys tell the story of his own first-hand experience of anatomy. In 1663 Pepys attended a dissection at London's Surgeons' Hall, accompanied by a lecture on the kidneys. The lecture was followed by a lavish dinner with the surgeons; but afterwards Pepys could not resist his curiosity and returned to the empty hall to see the corpse more closely. It was, he recorded in his famous diary, the body of 'a lusty fellow, a seaman, that was hanged for robbery. I did touch the dead body with my bare hand: it felt cold, but methought it was a very unpleasant sight.' Perhaps Moxon's dedication was a bit of gentle mockery of Pepys' distaste.

2 Jehan Cousin

It's notable that Moxon included 'statuaries [sculptors], painters, etc.' among those who, he hoped, would find the book useful. The symbiotic relationship between art and anatomy, established in the sixteenth century, continued into the seventeenth. Although artists still relied primarily on books of surgical anatomy, a separate publishing genre was already emerging. Albrecht Dürer's *Vier Bücher von menschlicher Proportion* (*Four Books on Human Proportion*) was followed by *Livre de pourtraiture* (*Book of Portraiture*), first printed in 1595 and running to several editions throughout the following century.

Its author Jehan or Jean Cousin (*c.*1522–95) was the son of Jean Cousin (*c.*1490–1560), a contemporary of Dürer's with whom he is often compared. Cousin the Elder was a highly regarded painter, sculptor and engraver who taught his son so well that their work is often indistinguishable. In 1560 he published his own book, *Livre de perspective* (*Book of Perspective*), in the knowledge that his son was working on the companion volume.

Thirty-five years was a long time to wait, and Jehan Cousin died before he could see his work in print. But today *Livre de pourtraiture* is considered a classic of the genre. He drew on his father's skills in geometry (the Elder also worked in stained glass) to demonstrate the proportions of various figures viewed from three different directions. It showed his own skill as an artist and his understanding of the human body.

The anatomy is restricted to musculature, and the full title of *Livre de pourtraiture* outdoes Remmelin's in terms of defining its target market: *Livre de pourtraiture de maistre Jean Cousin peintre et geometrien tres-excellent. Contenant par une facile instruction, plusieurs plans et figures de toutes les parties separees du corps humain: ensemble les figures entieres, tant d'ho[m]mes, que de femmes, et de petits enfans: veues de front, de profil, et de dos, avec les proportions, mesures, et dima[n]sions d'icelles, et certaines regles pour racourcir par art toutes lesdites figures: fort utile et necessaire aux peintres, statuaires, architectes, orfeures, brodeurs, menuisiers, et generalement à tous ceux qui ayment l'art de peinture et de sculpture* may be translated as *Very Excellent Portrait Book by Jean Cousin Painter and Geometrician. Containing Several Easy-to-use Plans and Figures of All the Separate Parts of the Human Body: together the Whole Figures, as Many Men, as of Women, and of Small Children: Seen from the Front, in Profile and Back, with the Proportions, Measures and Dimensions of These, and Certain Rules to Shorten all the Said Figures by Art: Very Useful and Necessary for Painters, Statuaries, Architects, Goldsmiths, Embroiderers, Carpenters and Generally for All Those who Love the Art of Painting and Sculpture.* In short, it's a book by an artist for artists.

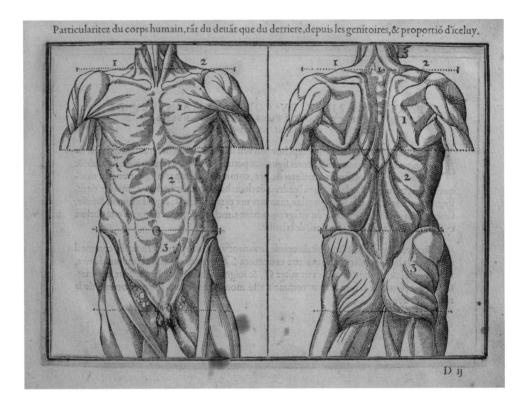

D ij

ABOVE

Livre de pourtraiture (1595)

Jehan Cousin's study book for artists, here illustrating the muscles of the torso. The publication was a companion to his father Jean Cousin's *Livre de perspective* (1560).

OPPOSITE

Anatomices et chirurgiae (1624)

Title page of a posthumous compilation of the works of Girolamo Fabrici, containing his tracts on the formation of the foetus, on speech, on animal sounds and on veins, with illustrations of foetus, tongue and a dissection.

3 Girolamo Fabrici

For anatomists, Padua continued to be the centre of excellence. The professorship held by Vesalius, Colombo and Falloppio passed to Falloppio's student Girolamo Fabrici (1533–1619), who designed the world's first anatomy theatre at the University of Padua. Three of Fabrici's students made important contributions to the subject in the seventeenth century and two of them succeeded him in his post.

Apart from his ample skills as a teacher, Fabrici was a prolific author of medical texts – around twenty in all. One of his early interests was in the development of the foetus, and by 1600 he had written both *De formatione ovi et pulli* (*On the Formation of the Egg and the Chicken*) and *De formato foetu* (*On the Formed Foetus*). The former no doubt raised the age-old question, 'Which came first?' He became fascinated by vocal sounds, and in 1603 he published first *De brutorum loquela* (*On the Speech of Animals*) and then *De locutione et eius instrumentis* (*On Speech and its Instruments*).

Ten years later Fabrici had broadened his scope with *Tractatus anatomicus triplex* (*Triple Anatomical Treatise*) which dealt with the eyes, the ears and the larynx. Before his death he had added papers on the muscles, the skeleton, breathing and the lungs, tumours, the digestive system from throat through stomach to intestines, the skin, and the mechanics of walking. Although Fabrici never published a single all-encompassing volume of anatomy, these individual treatises added up to a lifetime of investigation.

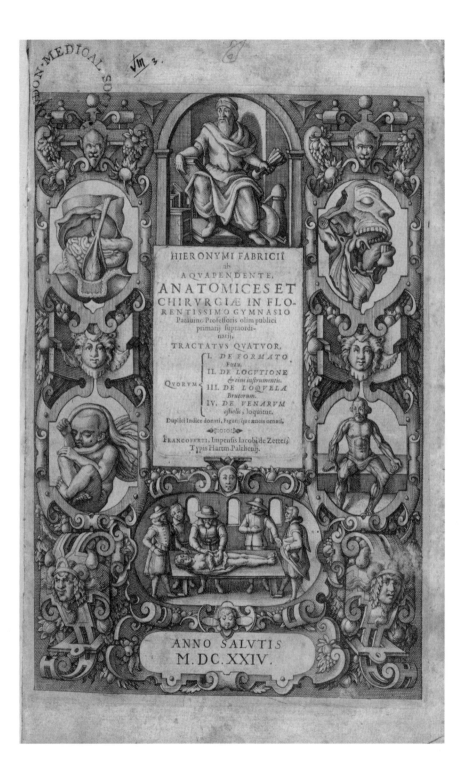

HIERONYMI FABRICII
ab
AQVAPENDENTE,
ANATOMICES ET
CHIRVRGIÆ IN FLO-
RENTISSIMO GYMNASIO
Patauino Professoris olim publici
primarij supraordi-
narij,
TRACTATVS QVATVOR,

QVORVM
{
I. DE FORMATO
Fœtu.
II. DE LOCVTIONE
& eius instrumentis.
III. DE LOQVELA
Brutorum.
IV. DE VENARVM
ostiolis, loquitur.
}

Duplici Indice donati, Figuris que æneis ornati.

FRANCOFVRTI, Impensis Iacobi de Zetter,
Typis Hartm. Palthenij.

ANNO SALVTIS
M.DC.XXIV.

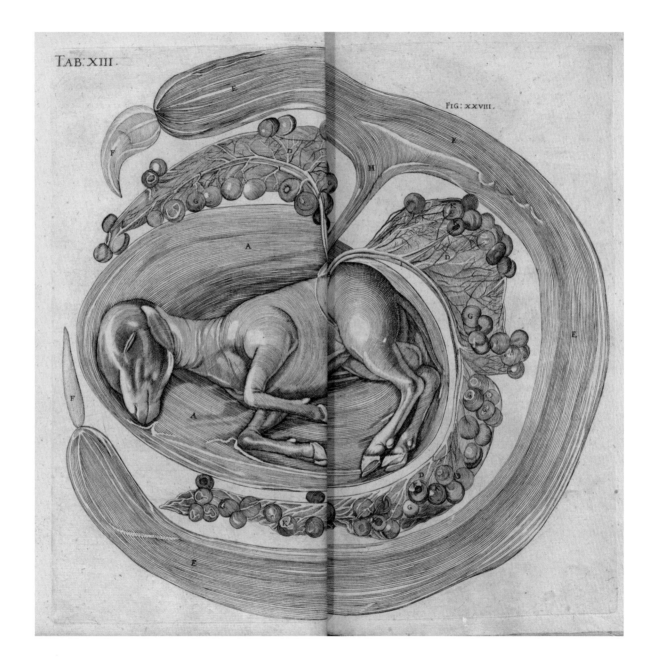

Girolamo Fabrici

Opposite: An ovine foetus in
the womb. Below left: The
organs of human speech.
Below: The veins of the
upper leg.

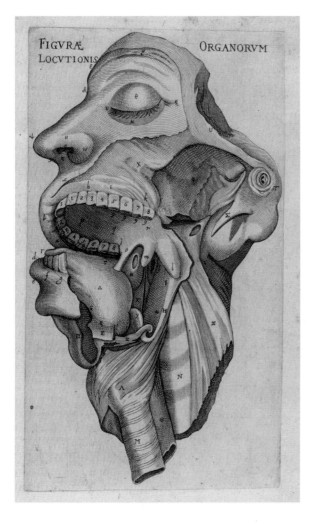

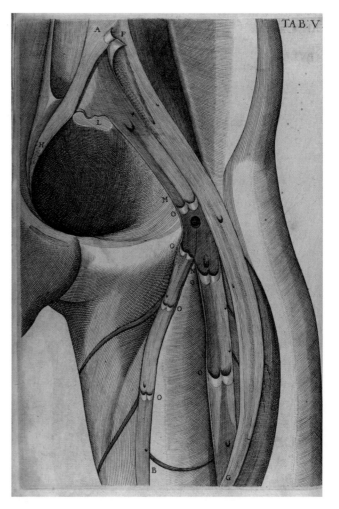

Right: A human foetus in the womb. Opposite: The development of a chicken in the egg.

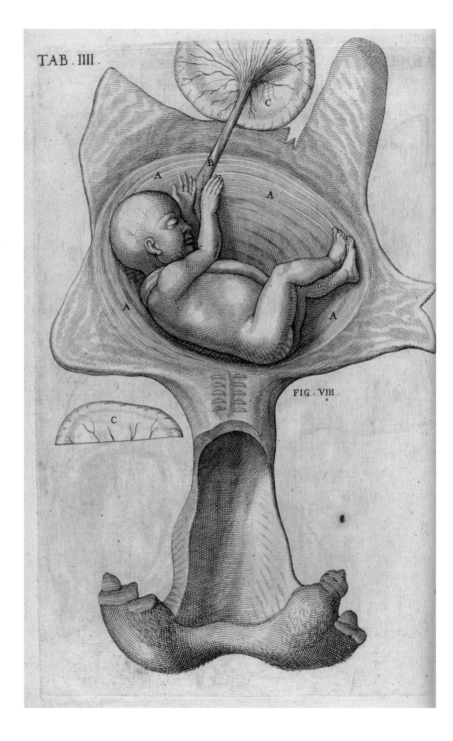

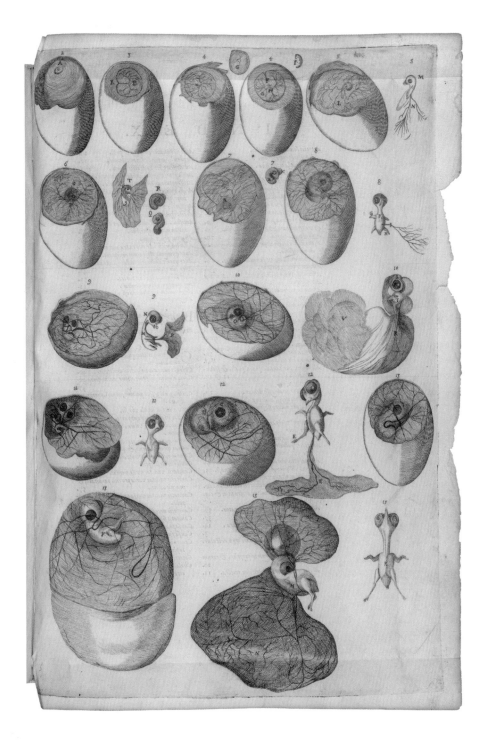

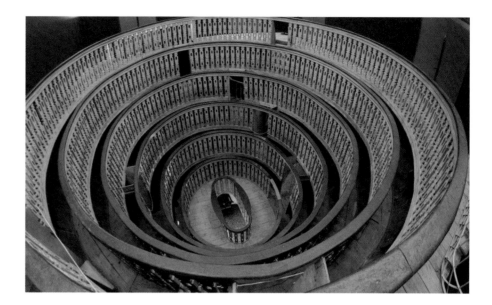

He worked principally from animal dissections but did not make unconfirmed assumptions about the human body. He was a skilled and experienced surgeon, and devised a procedure for tracheotomy which is similar to the one practised in today's hospitals.

4 Giulio Casseri and Adriaan van den Spiegel

Fabrici was a formidable anatomist and teacher. His curiosity was infectious, and his greatest legacy was to pass it on to his students. Giulio Casseri and Adriaan van den Spiegel studied alongside each other under him. Casseri succeeded Fabrici in the Chair of Medicine, and Spiegel succeeded Casseri. Their most important publications came out within a year of each other, and even shared the same illustrations.

Casseri (1552–1616) first came under the influence of Fabrici when, as a young man, he found work as a servant in the Fabrici household. When Casseri showed interest in Fabrici's work, the master took it upon himself to teach him privately. Casseri published *De vocis auditusque organis historia anatomica* (*The Anatomical History of the Voice and Organs of Hearing*) in 1601, fully two years before Fabrici's own books on voice, and perhaps prompted his teacher to visit the same subject. Like Fabrici, Casseri considered the mechanisms of sound in both animals and humans. Now that anatomists understood that there was a difference between animals and humans, the subject of comparative anatomy was ripe for development. Fabrici and Casseri were quick off the mark.

Casseri prepared corpses for dissection, and showed such promise as an anatomist that he took over teaching duties when Fabrici was unavailable. Much to Fabrici's irritation, Casseri, with the advantages of youth and lack of responsibility, proved far more popular with his students than the professor could hope to be; Fabrici promptly barred Casseri from any private teaching. When Fabrici withdrew from lecturing, the university

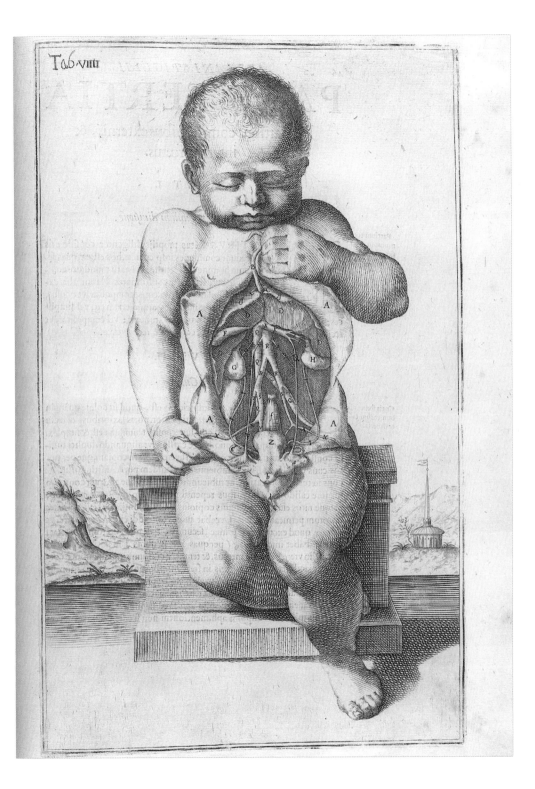

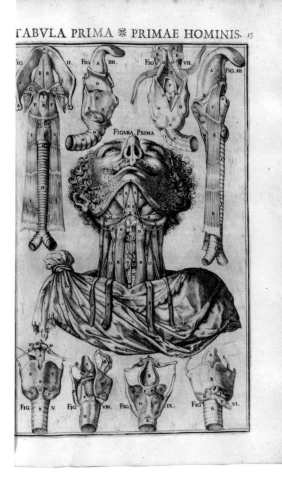

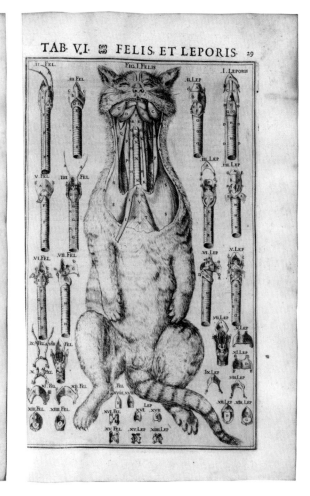

TAB· V.I· ❈ FELIS, ET LEPORIS· 29

Tabulae anatomicae (1627)

Giulio Casseri's illustrations finally saw the light of day in a book
written by his successor Adriaan van den Spiegel and edited by Daniel
Rindfleisch. From left to right: A detailed view of the anatomy of the
neck; comparative anatomies of the neck of a cat (*Felis*) and rabbit
(*Leporis*); details of the musculature surrounding the larynx; views of
a laryngotomy, with the surgical tools required for it.

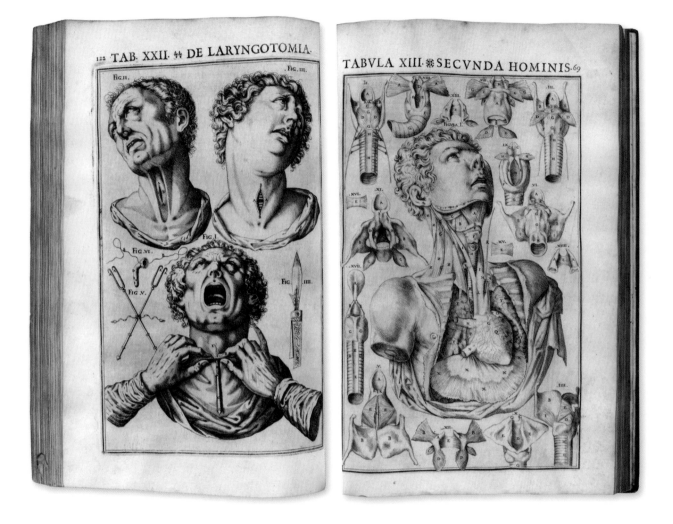

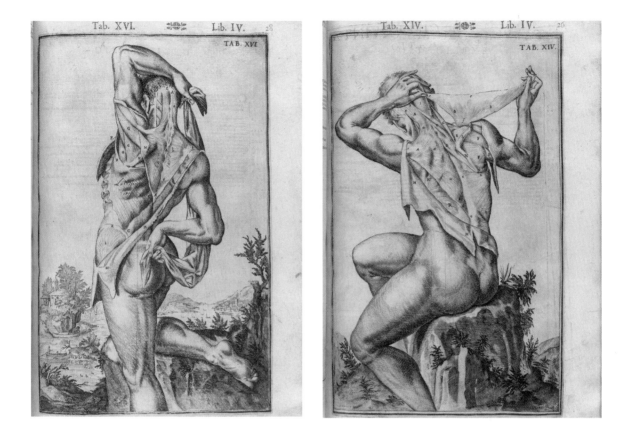

Casseri's artistry is evident not only in his anatomy but in the poses and undissected areas of his models' bodies, here displaying the muscles of their arms, legs and upper backs.

appointed Casseri as his successor – despite Fabrici's protests. But within weeks of his first public demonstration Casseri died of a fever.

He was a gifted artist and by the time of his death he had completed ninety-seven plates of anatomical illustrations intended for a grand atlas of the human body. After Adriaan van den Spiegel (1578–1625) succeeded him as Professor of Anatomy, the plates came into his possession and he planned his own book using Casseri's images. Spiegel was, like Vesalius, a native of the Low Countries and he intended his book to be both a tribute to and a revision of that great man's work. It was even to have the same title, *De humani corporis fabrica*. However, he too died before he could complete the project.

The plates then passed to Spiegel's son-in-law, who edited and published an old manuscript of Spiegel's, *De formato foetu* (*On the Formed Foetus*) in 1626, using some of Casseri's illustrations (and the title of Fabrici's 1600 work). The following year a German surgeon, Daniel Rindfleisch (sometimes known as Bucretius, the Latinised version of his name), edited and annotated Spiegel's notes for *De humani corporis fabrica* and published them in Venice under the title *Tabulae anatomicae* (*Anatomical Charts*).

The book must be regarded as a work of joint authorship by both Casseri and Spiegel, and including Rindfleisch, without whom neither of the other men's greatest work would have seen the light of day. A little later it was combined with *De formato foetu* in a single volume, and today *Tabulae anatomicae* is regarded as a major work of seventeenth-century anatomy.

It contains ninety-seven of Casseri's plates, engraved on copper by Francesco Valesio after works of Odoardo Fialetti, a pupil of Venice's greatest Renaissance painter, Tintoretto. They mark the pinnacle of the engraver's art, just as Vesalius's woodblocks did for the carver's skill a hundred years earlier. The book led the field for the rest of the century, and Casseri's images were copied for countless lesser works well into the next.

They are extraordinary images, accurate and uncluttered, elegant and playful. Each dissected figure, male or female, stands in a minimal landscape, with little enough detail to leave the focus on the body but enough to entertain the wandering eye – a ship by a river or a botanically correct plant species. Where skin is shown peeled back to reveal organs, it is artfully shown, as the petals of a flower around the revelation of the female reproductive system, for example. A sleeping baby holds the flaps of its skin as if they were its blanket and even a skeleton obligingly pulls a last shred of its skin out of the way to afford the viewer a better look.

Casseri and Spiegel both left their mark on anatomy. Spiegel lives on in: Spiegel's lobe, part of the liver; in the Spigelian line and the Spigelian fascia within the abdominal muscle group; and he described a rare abdominal injury, now known as a Spigelian hernia. Casseri, unlucky to have died before his work was presented to the world, also had the misfortune to have someone else's name attached to his discovery of the arterial circle in the brain; it is now called the Circle of Willis after English physician Thomas Willis who rediscovered it later in the century.

5 William Harvey

Padua attracted students from all over Europe. Among Fabrici's doctoral students from 1599 to 1602 was an Englishman, William Harvey. Harvey (1578–1657) graduated in the arts from the University of Cambridge before attending Fabrici's lectures at Padua. Fabrici recognised his keen mind and, for his part, Harvey admired Fabrici's work; he is known to have read Fabrici's *De venarum ostiolis* (*On the Gates of the Veins*), published the year after Harvey received his doctorate. That treatise described the membranous folds in veins for the first time, which Fabrici referred to as valves; but because of gaps in anatomical knowledge at the time he could not fully understand their function. We know now that they prevent blood from flowing in the wrong direction when it should be on its way back to the heart.

After passing his final exams *cum laude*, Harvey returned to Cambridge where he became qualified as a Doctor of Medicine. He found work in St Bartholomew's Hospital, a paupers' institution where he rose to become Physician in Charge. The charter there required him 'to do the best of your knowledge in the profession of physic to the poor then present, or any other of the poor at any time of the week which shall be sent home unto you by the Hospitaller.'

He maintained his connection with St Bartholomew's for almost the whole of his life; but it was not well paid and consisted chiefly of writing prescriptions for medicines. It

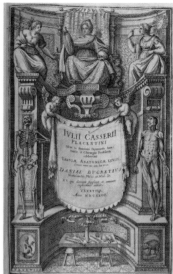

ABOVE
Tabulae anatomicae (1627)

Among the images on the title page are a skeleton with a spade, a flayed man and a table bearing the tools of the anatomist's trade.

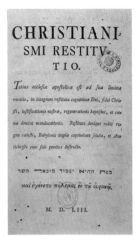

ABOVE
Christianismi restitutio (1553)

The radical Christian doctrine
in Miguel Servet's book
overshadowed his discovery
of the circulation of blood in
the body.

RIGHT
*An Anatomical Account
of the Motion of the Heart
and Blood* (1628)

An illustration of William
Harvey's experimental
proof, using ligatures, of the
difference between veins and
arteries.

made relatively small demands on his aptitude for anatomy, although it may have
provided opportunities for him to practice it on the corpses of patients whom he was
unable to save. In 1615, however, his career received a significant boost when he was
appointed as the Lumleian Lecturer. The Lumley Lectures, named after the man, Baron
Lumley, who originally endowed them, were established in 1582 as a means of promoting
anatomical knowledge among England's medical profession. One of the oldest
continuously running lecture series in the world, the Lumley Lecture is still presented
annually by the Royal Society of Physicians.

It was during his first season of Lumley Lectures, in 1616, that Harvey made the first
announcement of the discovery for which he is famous. In doing so, he resolved the
problem that had defeated anatomists from the very start: where does blood come from,
and where does it go? Harvey had uncovered what many of his predecessors had come
very close to: the body's circulation system. In the thirteenth century, Ibn al-Nafis had
been the first to propose a sort of pulmonary circulation, challenging Galen's belief in two
separate systems of blood and pneuma. Galen's theory persisted, nevertheless, until and
beyond Harvey's publication of his ideas, although others had come close to the truth,
among them Colombo, Vesalius and da Vinci.

Over the following twelve years he was able to confirm and develop his theory, which
he published at last in 1628 as *Exercitatio anatomica de motu cordis et sanguinis in
animalibus* (*An Anatomical Account of the Motion of the Heart and Blood in Animals*).
Over seventy-two pages Harvey explained his inescapable conclusion while refuting the
theories of others. Of the notion that blood was produced in the liver, for example, as
embraced by Galenists, he was scathing. If the heart pumps out around 20cc (⅙fl oz)
with each beat, and if it beats 2,000 times an hour, then every hour it delivers 9.4kg
(20lb 6oz). Every day the liver would have to produce 225.9kg (498lb) of blood, much
more than twice the entire bodyweight of the average Englishman.

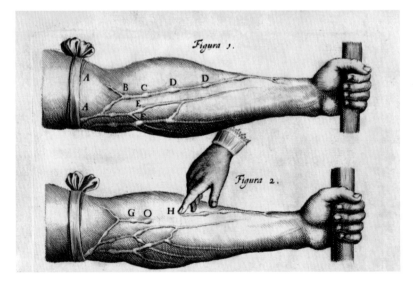

Instead of tackling the question of whether or not the heart was the seat of the soul, Harvey considered the body from a purely mechanical perspective. The heart was a pump, not a temple; the blood vessels carried blood, not pneuma, to and from the heart; and the pulses in them were caused by the contractions of the heart, not by themselves. His approach was scientific, empirical and analytical. He dissected animals of all kinds and used what he found there to form and test theories about human circulation.

He found that the left and right ventricles worked together, not independently as previously thought. As the possibility of circular flow began to present itself, he did further experiments, first on animals and then on humans. If he tied off the veins, the heart became empty; if he tied off the arteries, the heart swelled up. By tying a ligature to a human arm, he observed that the lower arm became pale and cold; by loosening it a little the arm reddened and heated up, because pressure on the arteries, which lie deeper in the arm, had been relieved. In causing the veins to bulge, Harvey was able to see little bulges within them, which were the valves discovered by his mentor Fabrici; valves were evidence of a one-way system, which he confirmed by trying to force blood backwards through the veins. Harvey's book is admired as much for his process as for his discovery.

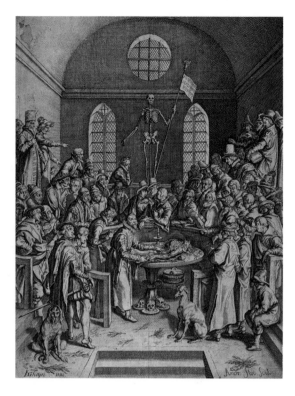

ABOVE

Succenturiatus anatomicus (1616)

An early monograph focussing on a single organ – the brain. The author Pieter Pauw is pictured in the frontispiece delivering an anatomy lesson in an engraving by Andries Stock after Jacques de Gheyn. The venue is the anatomy theatre in Leiden which Pauw built.

One man did beat Harvey to it. A Spaniard, Miguel Servet (*c*.1509–53), wrote in 1553 that 'the blood is passed through the pulmonary artery to the pulmonary vein for a lengthy pass through the lungs, during which it becomes red, and gets rid of the sooty fumes by the act of exhalation.' Unfortunately, the book in which he published this breakthrough was *Chriſtianismi reſtitutio* (*The Reſtoration of Chriſtianity*), a rejection of the fundamental Christian principles of Predestination and the Holy Trinity. For this, he was convicted of heresy and burnt alive on a pile of his own books; and his insights remained hidden from general view.

William Harvey anticipated resistance to his ideas, and he was not disappointed. As one biographer put it, many doctors would 'rather err with Galen than proclaim the truth with Harvey.' He feared not only 'injury to myself from the envy of a few, but I tremble lest I have mankind at large for my enemies . . . still the die is cast, and my trust is in my love of truth, and the candour that inheres in cultivated minds.' It took another twenty years for the idea of pulmonary circulation to win over medical minds, and hearts.

In order to gain maximum exposure for his work, Harvey printed *De motu cordis* in Frankfurt, which had been a centre of publishing since the twelfth century when handwritten manuscripts were exchanged in the city. An annual book fair established in Frankfurt in 1462 was (and still is) used as a testing ground for new ideas in print. Today

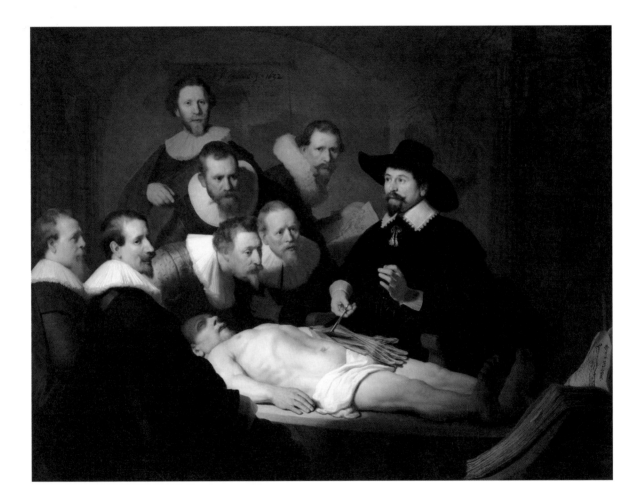

Frankfurt Book Fair is the largest such event in the world, and it certainly helped to disseminate Harvey's truth in 1628.

Harvey also identified the double circulation system in which blood returned to the heart is then circulated to the lungs before being sent around the body once more. There was one aspect of circulation which he was unable to prove by observation. Armed only with the naked eye and a magnifying glass, he could only theorise about capillaries, the web of tiny blood vessels – less than ten micrometers in diameter – which carry blood from the arteries to the veins.

The microscope was in its infancy in the early seventeenth century. The great astronomer Galileo Galilei patented the first compound (multi-lens) microscope in 1609 and is known to have manufactured one in 1624, only four years before Harvey published *De motu cordis*. The Netherlands was a centre for the production of lenses for eye pieces and much of the early development of microscopes took place there.

Thanks to the anatomy school in Leiden, Holland was already a centre of research. Leiden's anatomy theatre was only the second one in the world after Padua's, constructed in 1594; and the symbiosis between art and anatomy was as strong in northern Renaissance Europe as it was in the south. The walls of the anatomist's library are decorated with several paintings which illustrate the relationship. One crowded and animated engraving by Andries Stock (from an original drawing by Jacques de Gheyn) shows a demonstration in progress in the theatre at Leiden in 1615. It is being conducted by Pieter Pauw, a student under Fabrici who became Leiden's first Professor of Anatomy.

Most famously, Rembrandt (a native of Leiden) painted at least two scenes of dissection: *The Anatomy Lesson of Dr Nicolaes Tulp* (1632) and *The Anatomy Lesson of Dr Deijman* (1656). Tulp and Deijman were successive Amsterdam City Anatomists, and because – by law – they were only allowed one body a year for dissection it's possible to date the scenes and identify the corpses precisely. Dr Tulp is shown dissecting the cadaver of Aris Kindt, who was hanged for armed robbery on 31 January 1632. The large book at the corpse's feet is the same size and shape as Vesalius's *De humani corporis fabrica*. Dr Deijman's armed robber, Joris 'Black Jan' Fonteijn, was hanged on 29 January 1656. Rembrandt's use of shortened perspective in this painting draws the viewer into the presence of the dissection.

6 Giovanni Battista Hodierna, Jan Swammerdam and Marcello Malpighi

Despite this Dutch excellence in anatomy, art and the manufacture of lenses, the earliest book to show microscopic anatomical images came not from the Netherlands but from Sicily. Worse, it was written not by an anatomist but by an astronomer. Giovanni Battista Hodierna (1597–1660) published *L'occhio della mosca* (*The Eye of the Fly*) in 1644. He was a priest who studied the night sky in his spare time until he was appointed as astronomer to Giulio Tomasi, Duke of Palma. His many important contributions to that science, published mostly in Palermo, were overlooked and forgotten until their rediscovery in 1985. Anatomy was a relatively minor interest, and in the same year as *L'occhio della mosca* he wrote a treatise on weights and measures and their use in detecting impure gold and silver.

OPPOSITE

The Anatomy Lesson of Dr Nicolaes Tulp (1632)

Rembrandt's painting of the Amsterdam city anatomist Dr Tulp dissecting the body of a man, Aris Kindt, who had been hung for armed robbery.

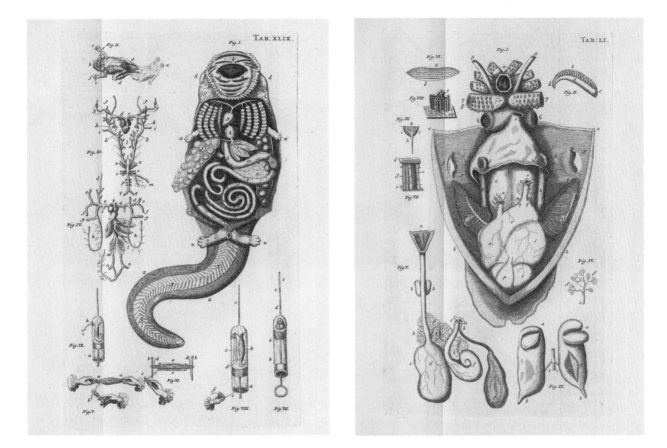

Published long after his
death, Jan Swammerdam's
microscopic studies of animal
anatomy were a revelation.
Left: A tadpole, below which
are Swammerdam's experiments
in muscle contraction. Right:
Swammerdam's dissection of a
cuttlefish.

Microscope anatomy was principally seen as a novelty by the book-buying public, but
anatomists themselves gradually began to see its possibilities. Jan Swammerdam (1637–
80), a Dutch graduate from the University of Leiden, was a pioneer in the field. His early
studies were in the life cycles of insects and his *Bybel der natuure* (*Bible of Nature*),
published only in 1737 long after his death, was a comprehensive insect anatomy
observed by dissection and microscope. He saw his work as a tribute to the wonders of
God, whose supremacy he saw in even the smallest creature. Of one unregarded beast, for
example, he wrote: 'Herewith I offer you the Omnipotent Finger of God in the anatomy
of a louse: wherein you will find miracle heaped on miracle and see the wisdom of God
clearly manifested in a minute point.' In the human sphere, Swammerdam was the first
man to see red blood cells through a microscope, in 1658.

Swammerdam's microscopic enquiries were driven by the availability of instruments and
the research of an Italian microbiologist, Marcello Malpighi (1628–94). Malpighi studied
anatomy at Bologna but was as fascinated by plants and insects as by human bodies. His
Anatome plantarum (*Anatomy of the Plants*), published in two volumes between 1675 and
1679, sits alongside his *De pulmonis epistolae* (*A Letter about the Lungs*).

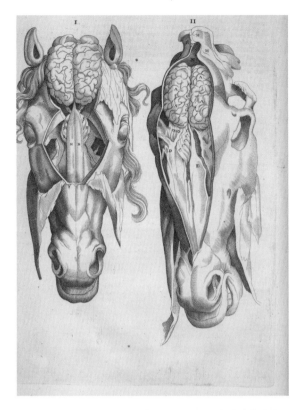

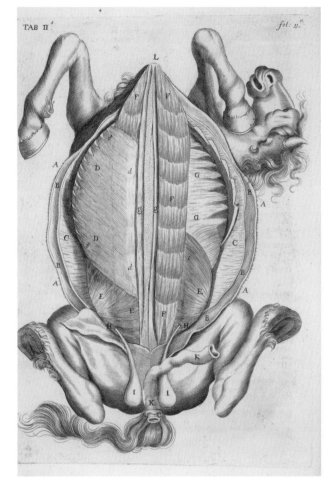

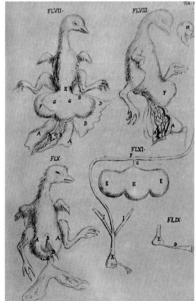

LEFT

De formatione de pulli in ovo (1673)

Marcello Malpighi made a series of very detailed studies of the formation of the embryo of a chick inside an egg.

ABOVE

The Anatomy of an Horse (1683)

Andrew Snape's book drew on the sixteenth-century work of Carlo Ruini, with new plates by the English engraver Robert White. Left: Anatomy of the equine skull and brain. Right: Muscles of the belly of a horse.

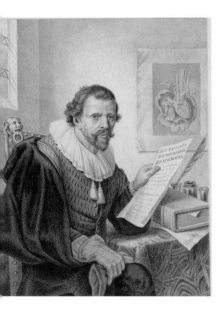

He made several discoveries about both the lungs and the body's waste disposal systems (many of which bear his name – for example, the Malpighian corpuscles and pyramids in the kidneys); but he was proudest of *Anatome plantarum*, illustrated by English engraver Robert White, which he later described as 'the most elegant format in the whole literate world.' White was best known for his portraiture of English nobility, but also executed some notable anatomical images. His work also illustrates John Browne's *A Compleat Discourse of Wounds* (1678), a manual in the tradition of the *wundarzt*; and Andrew Snape's *The Anatomy of an Horse* (1683), drawing on the sixteenth-century engravings of Carlo Ruini.

It was in the course of Malpighi's research on the lungs of animals that he made his greatest contribution to human anatomy. In the wake of Harvey, he investigated pulmonary circulation. He began by injecting black ink into the blood of sheep, to follow its course. But, like Harvey, he could not see what happened between the arteries and veins – even with the magnification at his disposal, the capillaries were too small to see. His breakthrough came in 1661 (just a year after Harvey's death) when he dissected a frog, in which the capillaries of the lungs were – at last – large enough to be seen with a microscope. This momentous discovery confirmed Harvey's hypothesis of a closed circulatory system, and Malpighi published his findings that year in *De pulmonibus observationes anatomicae* (*Anatomical Observations of the Lungs*).

The summit of Malpighi's investigations into blood was his 1666 work *De polypo cordis* (*The Polyp in the Heart*). It too owed much to the microscope, through which he made significant discoveries about the nature of blood clots, their formation and their difference in the left and right ventricles of the heart. Unaware of Swammerdam's work, he also observed red blood cells (and was the first into print about them). Malpighi requested that after his death (from a stroke) his body be submitted for an autopsy, one of the first instances of a body being willingly donated to medical science.

7 Charles Scarborough, Thomas Willis, Robert Hooke and Sir Christopher Wren

It is possible that Sir Christopher Wren, the architect of St Paul's Cathedral in London, met William Harvey, who spent a brief period teaching at the University of Oxford in the 1640s. Wren (1632–1723) is less well known for his experiences as an anatomist than as an architect; but he was instructed in the former by a pupil of Harvey's, Charles Scarborough, and for a while became Scarborough's assistant in dissections. Scarborough (1615–94) wrote *Syllabus musculorum* (*Syllabus of the Muscles*), a book of muscular anatomy which was a standard teaching text for many years, and succeeded Harvey as Lumleian Lecturer. Wren, like all university students before and since, viewed his university years as a time in which strong friendships were formed and he is the thread connecting several great anatomists of the age.

Wren was a member of the Oxford Philosophical Society, a group of enquiring scientific minds which included the groundbreaking chemist Robert Boyle and the anatomist Thomas Willis. Willis (1621–75) was one of the physicians who treated Anne

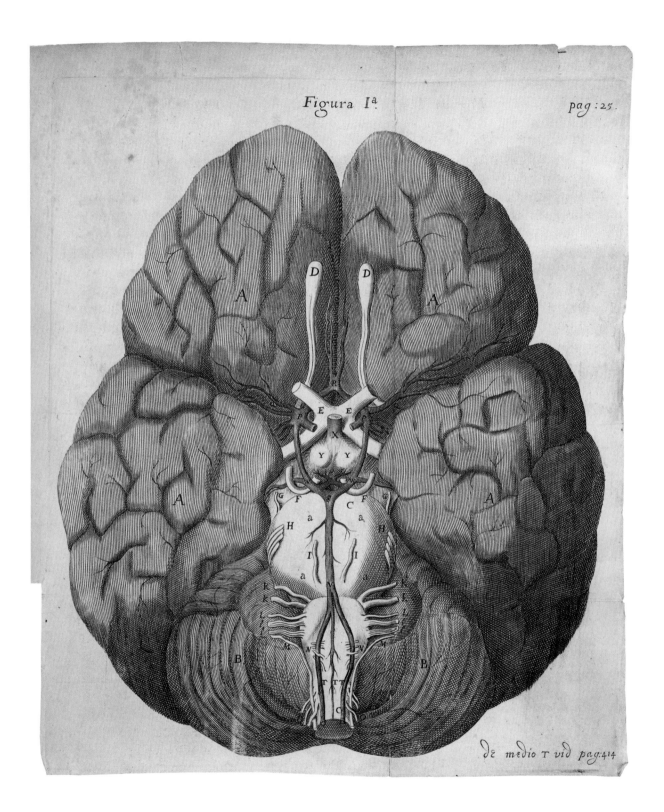

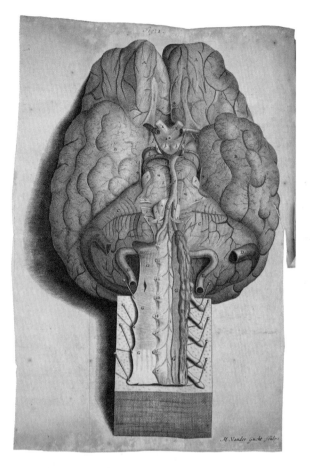

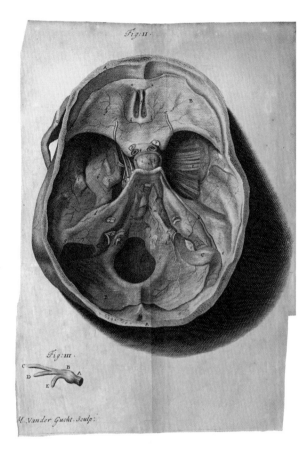

Greene, a woman whose survival after her hanging for infanticide in 1650 was regarded
as an act of divine intervention. (To emphasise God's position in the matter, her
prosecutor Sir Thomas Read had died three days after her failed execution.) Her sentence
was repealed, and the case became a sensational news story which made Willis's name.

When it came to dissection, Willis preferred to study the brains of recently hanged
criminals; the method of execution, he observed, resulted in swollen blood vessels within
the head which could more easily be seen. He also injected vessels with quicksilver or
coloured wax to make them more visible, and as a result was the first anatomist to
describe several features of the brain, including the vitally important blood-brain barrier.

Willis made a detailed study of the brain and the nervous system, which he published
in 1664 as *Cerebri anatome* (*The Anatomy of the Brain*). It is a marvel of a book,
meticulous and complex in its descriptions, far in advance of any preceding work on the
subject. It earned Willis a reputation as the father of neurology, a word which he coined
in his book. *Cerebri anatome* contains a host of innovations, including Willis's rediscovery
of the Ring of Willis first identified by the unlucky Giulio Casseri. Willis also deserves

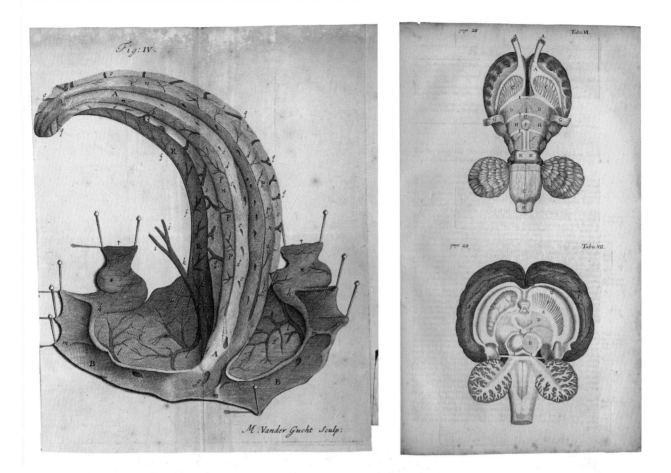

M. Vander Gucht Sculp:

recognition for his 1672 volume *Two Discourses concerning the Soul of Brutes, which is that of the Vital and Sensitive of Man*, which is regarded as the first English contribution to the science of medical psychology.

The illustrations in *Cerebri anatome* were by his friend Christopher Wren, and the book reflected Willis's collaborative work with another anatomist, Richard Lower. In some of those collaborations, Willis engaged the services of an assistant, Robert Hooke, who would go on to do great things in his own right.

Robert Hooke (1635–1703) later acted as an assistant to Willis's fellow Oxford Philosophical Society member Robert Boyle, who was also at the centre of the Invisible College of London, another group devoted to experimental science. In 1662 the members of both societies, with others, formed the Royal Society, under the patronage of Charles II, for the promotion and advancement of science. Members gave practical lectures on many branches of science and when the Society felt that the preparation of demonstrations justified a permanent appointment, Robert Boyle recommended Hooke for the post of Curator of Experiments. This not only gave Hooke experience of a wide

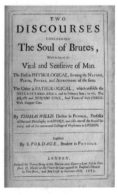

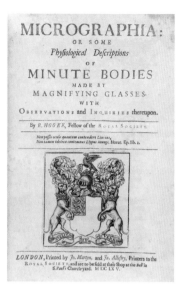

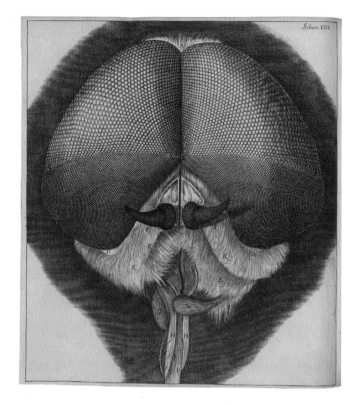

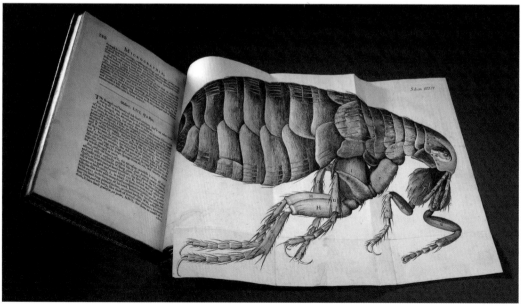

range of technologies but allowed him to present some of his own theories.

Hooke is one of many men regularly nominated for the accolade of England's Leonardo da Vinci. He was an extraordinary polymath who made great advances in many fields – heat, light, palaeontology, geology, gravity, mathematics and more. He applied mathematics to map-making and became London's Chief Surveyor, proposing a new grid plan for the city after it was destroyed by the Great Fire in 1666. He worked closely with Wren on the rebuilding of the city's churches and other buildings after the fire, and the engineering of the dome of St Paul's Cathedral is his. His experiments with respiration and combustion brought him close to the discovery of oxygen, while his microscopic examination of fossils anticipated the theory of natural evolution.

It was with the microscope that he made his greatest contribution to anatomy. *Micrographia*, which he published in 1665 only a year after his mentor Willis's *Cerebri Anatome*, is a treasure trove of illustrations of biology seen for the first time through a lens. It contains the first detailed views of tiny insects, on pages which fold out to emphasise the power of the microscope. The louse beloved of Jan Swammerdam, for example, unfolds in Hooke's book on a page four times larger than the book's cover. In studies of plants, Hooke observes the minute compartments of which they are composed, and names them 'cells' – the first use of the word in this context. *Micrographia* has the first ever image of a micro-organism, the microfungus Mucor. It is, in effect, a book of visual dissection, and when Hooke looks at fossilised wood and sees the same structures, he suggests an organic origin rather than the more fanciful explanations for fossils which were usually offered. Many images are presented in circular frames, giving viewers the sense of looking down a microscope at the objects in question.

Micrographia also includes microscope views of household objects such as pins and razor edges, and the whole book might have been passed off as an example of microscope novelty, had it not been published by the Royal Society. Instead, it was a mutually beneficial publication, boosting both Hooke's and the Society's scientific reputations.

In later life Robert Hooke fell out with Isaac Newton, a future president of the Royal Society, over whose theory about gravity came first. Hooke claimed to have given Newton the idea; and Newton is said to have hidden Hooke's papers and removed Hooke's portrait from the Society walls in revenge. No known portrait of Hooke survives.

The microscope which Robert Hooke used to prepare *Micrographia* was constructed by a London instrument maker, Christopher White. A true treasure of scientific history, it has survived to the present day and is displayed in the United States' National Museum of Health and Medicine in Maryland.

8 Antonie van Leeuwenhoek

This was a remarkable Golden Age of Science, when a profusion of ideas and discoveries tumbled from the minds of great men in England and the Netherlands. The Royal Society became a focal point for international cooperation; and, although he never wrote a book, there

OPPOSITE
Micrographia (1665)

Robert Hooke's celebrated book introduced microscopic images to the British public. Above left: The title page. Above right: The eye of a fly. Below: A giant louse unfolds from the pages, emphasising the power of microscopy.

BELOW
Robert Hooke's microscope

The lenses through which Hooke prepared *Micrographia* are preserved in the National Museum of Health and Medicine in Maryland, USA.

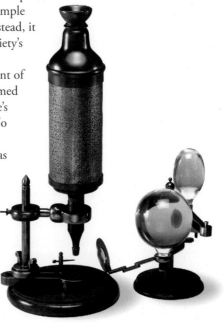

should be space on the library shelves for a bound volume of Antonie van Leeuwenhoek's correspondence with the Society, which later published them.

Van Leeuwenhoek (1632–1723) was a citizen of Delft in the Dutch Republic and spent his whole life there. He began his working life as an apprentice bookkeeper in a draper's shop, and the need to examine the quality of the cloth through a magnifying glass spurred his interest in lenses and microscopy. He made his own, over 500 in his lifetime, with magnification of up to 500x; and where other anatomists resorted occasionally to the microscope, van Leeuwenhoek's scientific work revolved entirely around the instrument. Even Robert Hooke, who had done so much for the microscope, was moved to complain that the field of microscopy was dominated by just one man – van Leeuwenhoek.

He was self-taught, and thought of his activities as no more than a hobby, of no interest to others. His thirst for microscopic views led to many discoveries; but they might have remained unknown to the world had his friend, the Dutch anatomist Reinier van Graaf, not written to the Royal Society in praise of van Leeuwenhoek's skill as a microscope-maker. Van Graaf's endorsement persuaded the Society to take Van Leeuwenhoek seriously; and in their next journal they published a letter from him sharing his microscopic observations of bees, lice and mould.

It became clear that he was skilled not only in the craft of manufacture but in the science of microscopy. Among his discoveries were: the existence of spermatozoa; a structure called a vacuole, which exists within cells to isolate dangerous or waste material; and a class of freshwater life forms which are neither plant, nor fungus, nor animal, known today as Protista. His observation of bacteria in the mouths of humans and other animals was of great importance. But, despite his many triumphs, the Society was suspicious when he wrote in 1676 that he had seen single-celled organisms. How could a single cell possibly function as an organism? So resistant to the idea were the members of the Society, and so insistent was Van Leeuwenhoek that they existed, that the Society dispatched a delegation to Van Leeuwenhoek's home to see for themselves. There, of course, they found the evidence, and in 1677 they acknowledged his discovery.

In 1680 he was elected a member of the Royal Society. Although he always shared his observations freely, Antonie van Leeuwenhoek was guarded about his process and especially about how he made his lenses. He worked alone and encouraged the idea that he ground all his lenses. The truth, that he fused thin glass rods in a flame, was only rediscovered in 1957, and it is now thought that Robert Hooke employed a similar method.

BELOW

Antonie van Leeuwenhoek (1632–1723)

A portrait by Dutch artist Jan Verkolje of the man known as the Father of Microbiology.

OPPOSITE

Neurographia universalis (1684)

A brain stripped of its meninges.

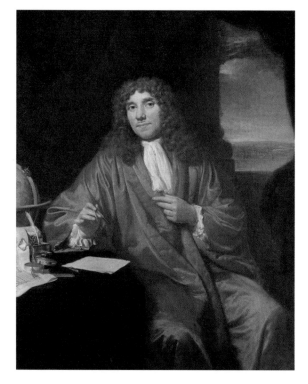

9 Raymond Vieussens and Humphrey Ridley

Thomas Willis's *Anatome cerebri* launched neurology as a new avenue for anatomical research. Before the end of the century at least two other notable anatomists had begun to build on his foundations. Raymond Vieussens, fourteen years Willis's junior, credited Willis with inspiring his career, which is noted for his work on the brain and the spinal cord. Vieussens (*c.*1635–1715) was the chief physician at the Hôtel Dieu Saint-Eloi hospital in Montpellier, the medical school at which he trained. He had a reputation during his life for indulging in speculation unsupported by the available scientific evidence. By freeing his imagination from the constraints of reality, he was able to consider new anatomical possibilities. That did not prevent his rigorous attention to detail in practice, and *Neurographia universalis* (*A Complete Neurology*), which he published in 1684, was a significant early work in the field of neurology, with some magnificent copperplate engravings as illustrations. For a while after its publication, the semi-oval mass of white matter below the cerebral cortex was known as Vieussens' centrum.

Vieussens also lent his name to several elements of the cardiovascular system, another field in which he took a great interest. One of his many publications was *Novum vasorum corporis humani systema* (*A New Vascular System of the Human Body*), printed in 1705 and an important early study of the anatomy and diseases of the heart which marks the beginnings of cardiology.

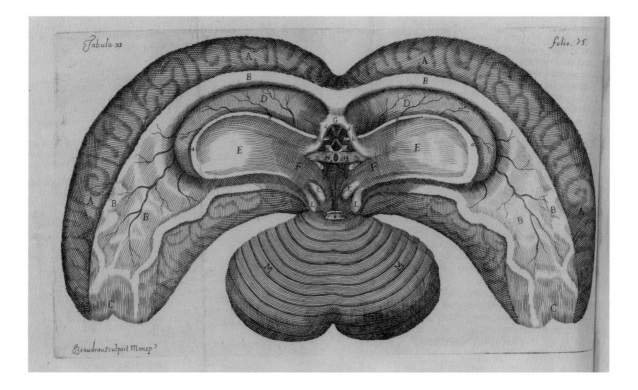

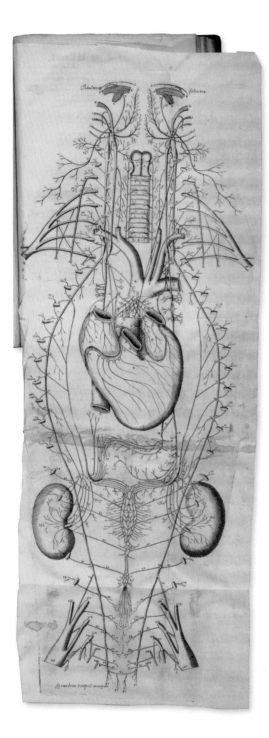

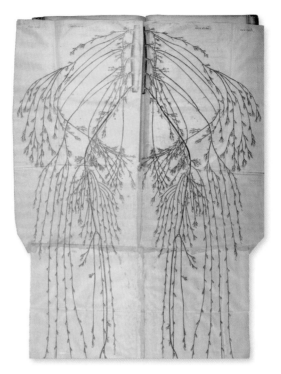

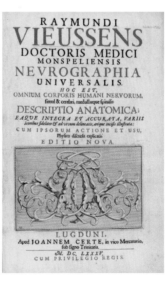

Neurographia universalis (1684)

Far left: Vieussens' overview of the central nervous system and its relationship with the heart, lungs, kidneys and spinal cord. Above: The spinal cord, the lumbosacral plexus and the nerves of the legs. Left: The title page of this early work of neurology.

Vieussens' exact contemporary, the English physician Humphrey Ridley, also picked up the baton left by Willis. Ridley (1653–1708) studied medicine in Leiden, where he graduated with a thesis on sexually transmitted diseases. But his most important publication is *The Anatomy of the Brain, containing its Mechanism and Physiology; together with some new Discoveries and Corrections of Ancient and Modern Authors upon that Subject*. It was a great advance in cerebral anatomy, and the first book of neurology to be published in English – Willis wrote in Latin. Largely forgotten today, Ridley made very important contributions in those early days of the science.

10 Reinier de Graaf, John Browne and William Molins

Reinier de Graaf (1641–73), Van Leeuwenhoek's sponsor at the Royal Society, published a number of anatomical works and made his own contributions to the science, especially concerning the reproductive system. He may have been the first man to identify the function of the Fallopian tubes, and the first man to describe the G-spot – although the 'G' stands for a later man, the gynaecologist Ernst Gräfenberg (1881–1957), who rediscovered it in the early twentieth century and also developed the IUD.

In 1668 De Graaf published *De virorum organis generationi inservientibus, de clysteribus et de usu siphonis in anatomia* (*On the Organs of Men which Serve for Generation, on Syringes and the Use of Siphons in Anatomy*). Some controversy arose from its 1672 sequel *De mulierum organis generationi inservientibus tractatus novus: demonstrans tam homines et animalia caetera omnia, quae vivipara dicuntur, haud minus quàm ovipara ab ovo originem ducere* (*A New Treatise on the Organs of Women which Serve for Generation: Showing Both Men and All Other Animals which are Called Viviparous, No Less than Oviparous, to Have their Origin from the Egg*). Fellow Dutchmen Jan Swammerdam and Johannes van Horne published the results of their own research *Miraculum naturae sive uteri muliebris fabrica* (*A Miracle of Nature or the Device of a Woman's Womb*) the same year; and Swammerdam accused De Graaf of plagiarising their discoveries concerning the uterus.

The accusation damaged De Graaf's reputation although he denied the charge; and elsewhere in his book he freely acknowledged that, for example, he had copied an illustration of an ectopic pregnancy from an earlier work. Whatever the truth, his work is a landmark in the history of reproductive anatomy, acting as a summary of all such knowledge to date but failing to advance it where it was flawed. For lack of human cadavers, he conducted most of his research on rabbits, and repeated several fallacies without checking either the original sources or the evidence of his own eyes. For example, he thought that fully formed humans were created in the ovary and simply brought to life and growth by the arrival of the spermatozoa.

A far worse example of plagiarism was committed by an English anatomist, John Browne, a few years later. In 1678 John Browne (1642–*c*.1702) published his competent *Compleat Discourse of Wounds*, with images by the same engraver, Chris White, who illustrated Marcello Malpighi's *Anatome plantarum*. Great things might have been expected of his next book *A Compleat Treatise of the Muscles as they Appear in the Humane Body and Arise in Dissection; with diverse anatomical observations not yet discovered*, which appeared in 1681.

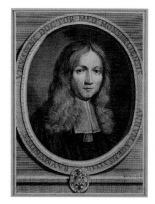

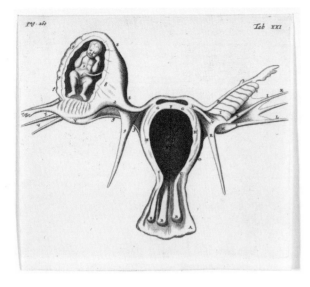

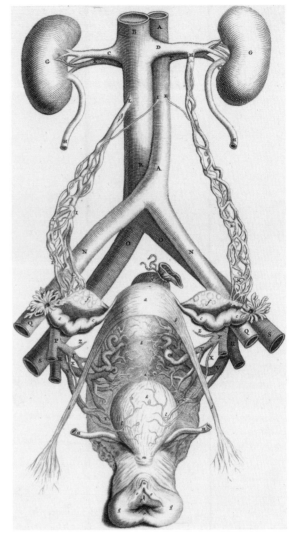

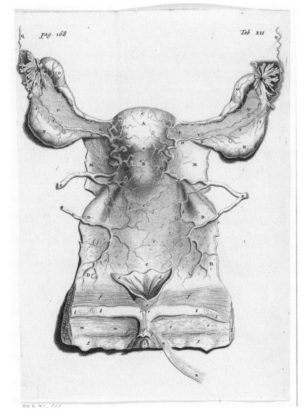

De mulierum organis generationi (1672)

Coinciding with a similar publication by Jan Swammerdam, Reinier de Graaf's work faced accusations of plagiarism. Left above: An image of ectopic pregnancy which De Graaf acknowledged having borrowed from an earlier book. Left: The interior of the uterus. Above: The female genitalia and urinary system.

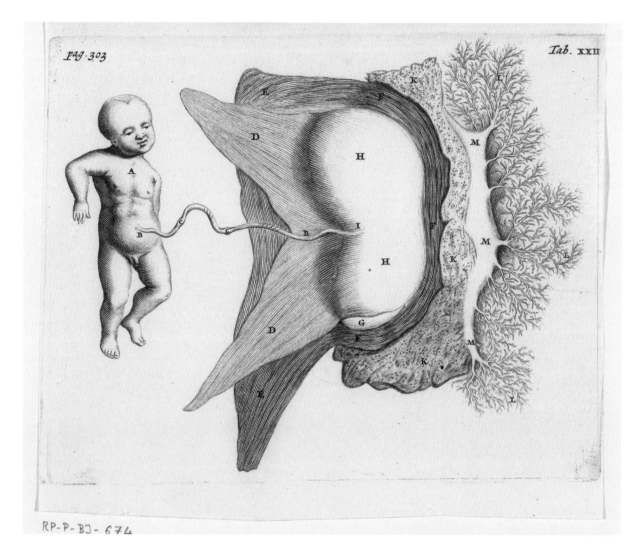

De mulierum organis generationi (1672)

A foetus attached by placenta to the womb. De Graaf's plates were etched by the highly regarded Dutch engraver Hendrik Bary.

John Browne plagiarised a text
by William Molins and images
by Giulio Casseri for his book
of 'anatomical observations
not yet discovered'. Left: The
muscles of the eyes and ears.
Right: The muscles of the neck.

Left: The muscles of the upper
torso, between the ribs. Right
above: The only original plate
in the book, a portrait of its
author John Browne. Right
below: The muscles of the
upper leg.

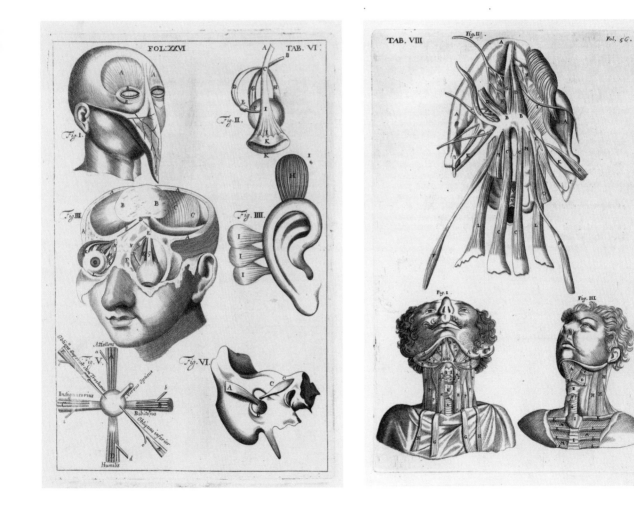

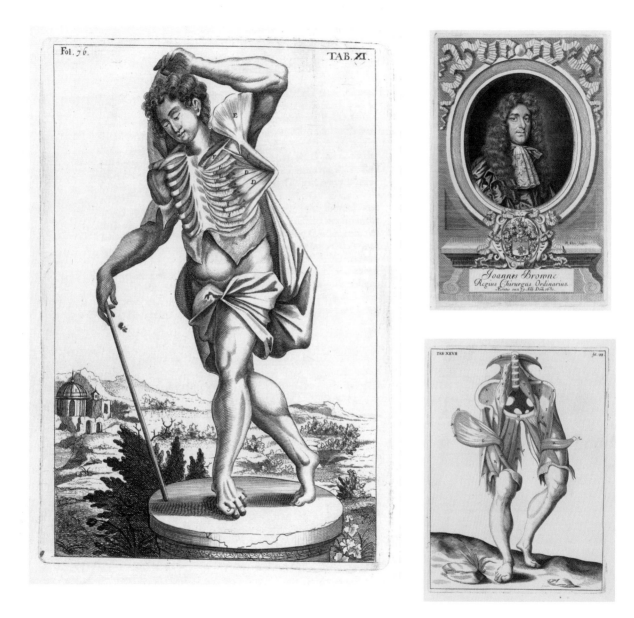

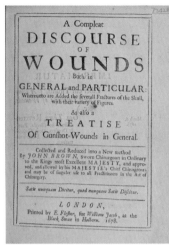

**A Compleat Discourse
on Wounds** (1678)

Above: Title page. Right:
Examples of fractures of the
skull. Opposite: A variety of
wounds on heads of all ages.

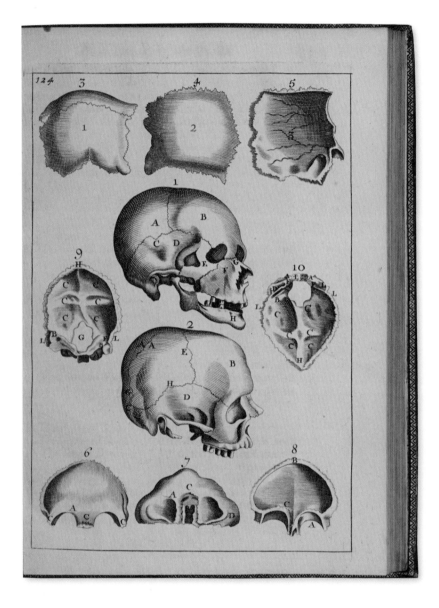

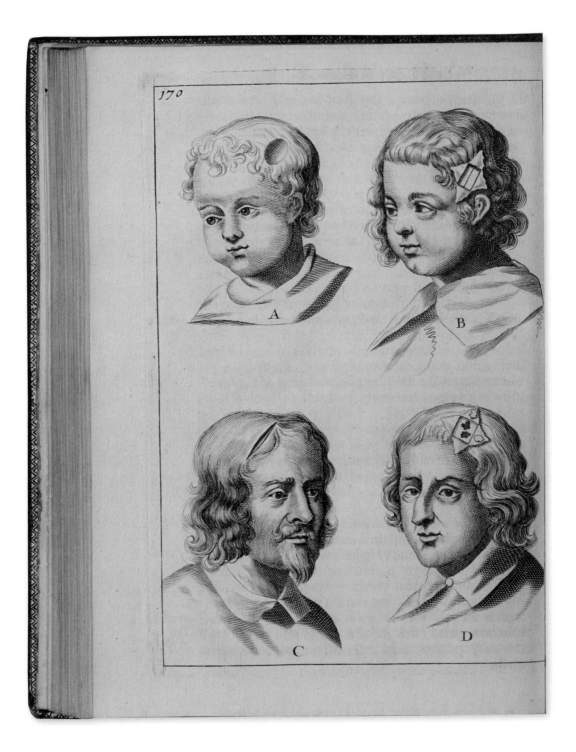

The title was misleading: the observations had in fact already been discovered – and published – by William Molins (1617–91) in 1648 as *Myskotomia, or The anatomical administration of all the muscles of an humane body, as they arise in dissection: as also an analitical table, reducing each muscle to his use and part; and published for the general good of all practitioners in the said art*. Browne had simply copied Molins' text; and to illustrate it he had used plates first published in Giulio Casseri's *Tabula anatomicae*.

Browne was exposed as a plagiarist in 1684, despite which the book sold well and ran to ten editions. He was later dismissed as a surgeon at St Thomas's Hospital in London for refusing to obey the hospital's regulations. Despite that, he was surgeon to two kings of England, Charles II and William III. Charles died in 1685 after several days of painful treatment from his doctors – including bloodletting, purging and cupping – following an apoplectic fit. William III outlived Browne by a few weeks.

11 Govert Bidloo and John Cowper

William III was Dutch, and his personal physician was another Dutchman, Govert Bidloo – who also suffered from plagiarism at the hands of an Englishman. Bidloo (1649–1713) was a literary man as well as an anatomist; he wrote plays and poetry, and in 1686 the libretto for Johan Schenck's *Bacchus, Ceres en Venus*, one of the first operas written by a Dutch composer (which, despite that, only premiered in 2011). A year before his libretto he wrote *Anatomia humani corporis* (*Anatomy of the Human Body*) which is notable for its 105 striking illustrations of human body parts drawn (both from the life and after dissection) by the artist Gerard de Lairesse and engraved by Abraham Blooteling. In it Bidloo described the papillary ridges on fingertips, and the book is chiefly remembered today for its contribution to solving crime through fingerprints.

Bidloo was appointed Professor of Anatomy at Leiden in 1695, and a year later he entered the service of William III. When the king died of pneumonia in 1702, it was in Bidloo's arms. A nephew of Bidloo's (Nicolaas Bidloo) later became the personal physician of the Russian Emperor, Peter the Great. Bidloo's book did not achieve the circulation its publishers hoped for, and to recoup their costs they sold off an overrun of 300 plates, either to an English publisher or to one of that publisher's authors – William Cowper. Cowper (1666–1709) was a gifted anatomist, remembered today in Cowper's gland, part of the male reproductive system. His 1694 book *Myotomia Reformata, or a New Administration of the Muscles*, led to his election as a member of the Royal Society in 1696.

Cowper's next book, *The Anatomy of Humane Bodies*, appeared in 1698 using the remaindered Bidloo plates throughout, without acknowledgement to either Bidloo or Lairesse. The frontispiece was identical too, except for a small piece of paper with Cowper's name and book title stuck over Bidloo's. Bidloo protested and a war of words ensued in which the two authors published tracts complaining of each other's behaviour. Cowper's defence, that he had bought the

BELOW

Anatomia humani corporis (1685)

The rather generic title page, in Dutch, of Govert Bidloo's lavishly illustrated book of anatomical detail.

OPPOSITE

Anatomia humani corporis (1685)

Left: A plate of eighteen figures showing blocks of skin, hair follicles and a fingertip. Right: The human eye at various stages of dissection.

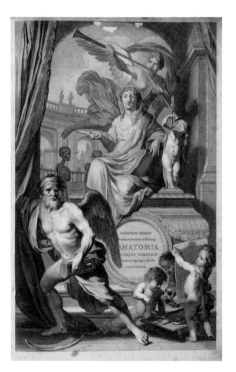

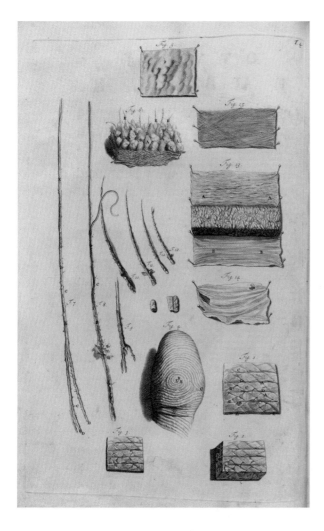

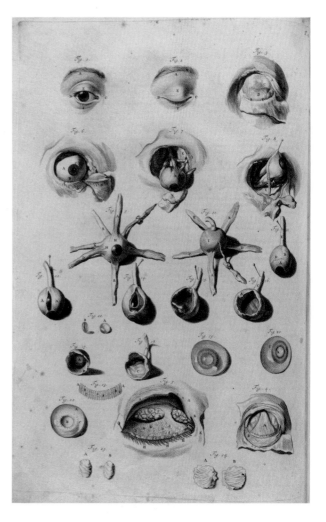

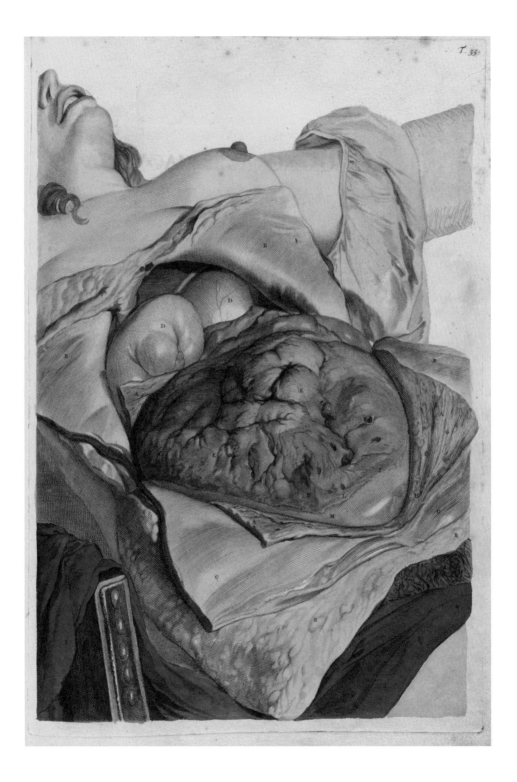

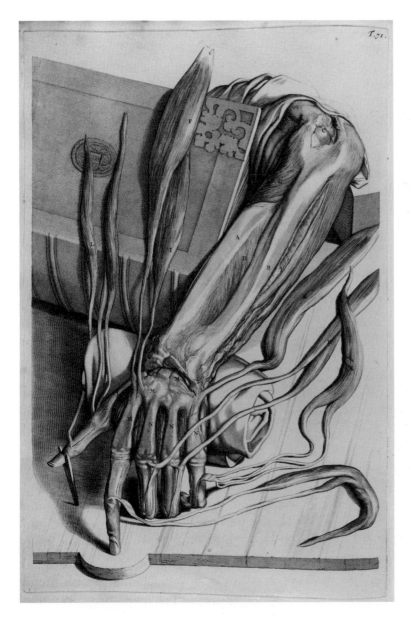

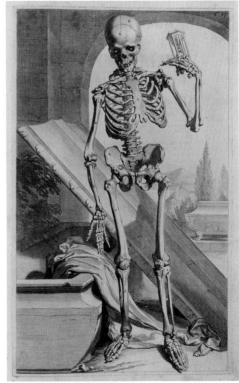

Anatomia humani corporis (1685)

Opposite: Bidloo's naturalistic, almost sensuous figures were engraved by Gerard de Lairesse. Left: Lairesse's imaginative presentation of the anatomy of the hand. Above: A skeleton holding a timer throws off its shroud and rises from the grave.

Right: The jaw and its muscles. Below: In contrast to the smiling figures of earlier anatomies, a twisted, écorché body exhibits muscles under tension.

Left: The muscles of the shoulder and face. Bidloo's images were determinedly unidealised. Right: William Cowper's English translation of Govert Bidloo's text gives the original author no credit on its title page.

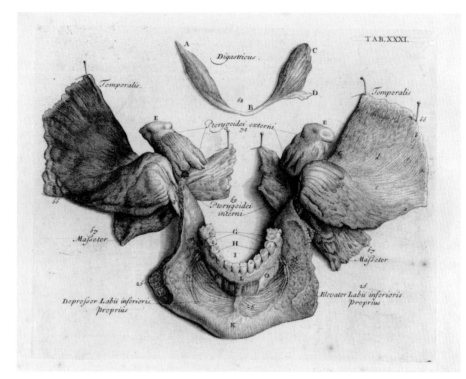

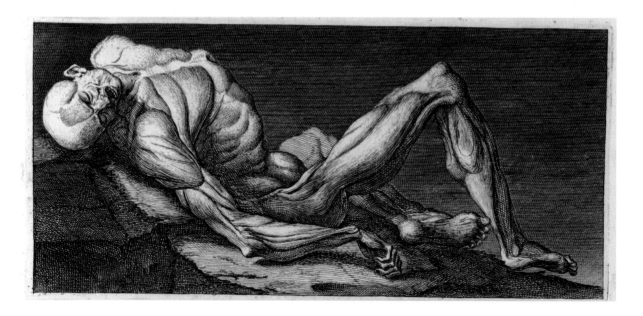

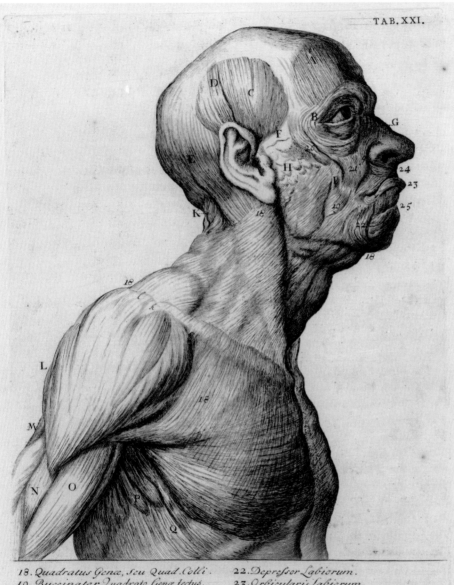

TAB. XXI.

MYOTOMIA REFORMATA:
OR AN
ANATOMICAL
TREATISE
ON THE
MUSCLES
OF THE
HUMAN BODY.
Illustrated with FIGURES after the LIFE.

By the late Mr. WILLIAM COWPER,
Surgeon, and Fellow of the Royal Society.

To which is prefix'd
An INTRODUCTION
CONCERNING
MUSCULAR MOTION.

LONDON:
Printed for ROBERT KNAPLOCK, and WILLIAM and JOHN INNYS,
in St. *Paul's Church-Yard*; and JACOB TONSON, in the
Strand. MDCCXXIV.

18. *Quadratus Genæ, seu Quad. Colli.*
19. *Buccinator Quadrato Genæ tectus.*
20. *Zygomaticus.*
21. *Elevator Labiorum.*

22. *Depressor Labiorum.*
23. *Orbicularis Labiorum.*
24. *Elevator labii superioris proprius.*
25. *Depressor labii inferioris proprius.*

The satirical English cartoonist Thomas Rowlandson (1757–1827) drew many caricatures of the medical profession. This one is said to have been inspired by the anatomy lectures of William Hunter.

plates from Jan Swammerdam's widow, was weak, especially in the light of the small piece of paper, and it implied that Bidloo was the plagiarist of Swammerdam's work.

Cowper did write an entirely new text to accompany them, full of interesting observations and new research; and he did expand the images, with nine new ones drawn by the English painter Henry Cooke and engraved by the Flemish artist Michiel van der Gucht. One might charitably argue that Cowper or his publisher simply made an error of omission in not crediting Bidloo's book as the source of the illustrations. Accidental or premeditated, Cowper's plagiarism has overshadowed his anatomy.

12 Edward Ravenscroft

Outside the scientific community, the public remained superstitiously opposed to dissection. There was a horror of meddling in something – the human body – which had, according to the Bible, been made in the image of God. It has long been a basis for humour that we laugh at the things which horrify or disgust us; and so, in the final years of the seventeenth century, a new comedy became a popular hit on the English stage. Edward Ravenscroft's bawdy farce *The Anatomist, or The Sham-Doctor* premiered in 1697. With the restoration of the monarchy, Charles II (who was having an affair with an actress) decreed that plays might be performed again (having been banned by Cromwell's republic) and that all female parts should be played by women (having previously been acted by men and boys).

Ravenscroft (1654–1707) is known in literary circles for being the first man to suggest that Shakespeare's *Titus Andronicus* was not written by William Shakespeare. In *The Anatomist* he wrote a creditable Shakespearean romantic comedy, with considerable emphasis on bodily functions and much intrigue among servants, masters and mistresses. It is still funny today, and as a historical record it sheds some light on the perception of anatomy at the time of its writing. One character, urged to visit the surgeon because there would be no risk in doing so, replies:

> No hazard, call you it? I hazard my legs, my arms, veins, arteries, and muscles; and in the Doctor's gibberish, I hazard incision, dissection, amputation, and circulation, thro' the systole and diastole. Why sir, in such a case, a physician cuts up a man with as little remorse, as a hangman carves a traitor.

No doubt there are many who fear a doctor's appointment today for the same reasons.

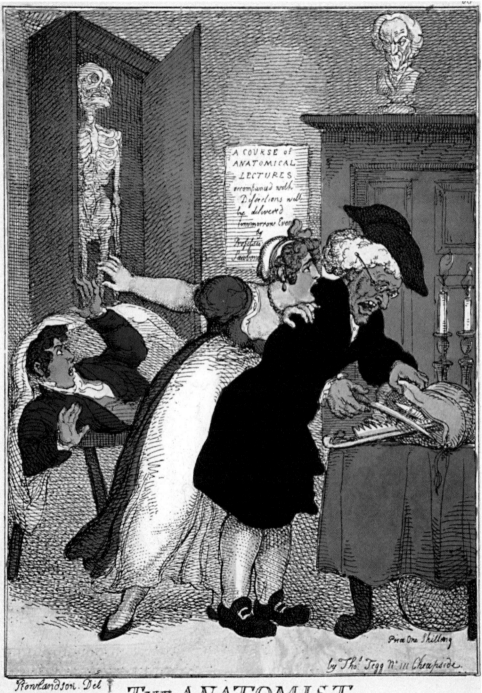

A COURSE of ANATOMICAL LECTURES accompanied with Dissections will be delivered Tomorrow Evening by Professor Sawbone

Prce One Shilling

by Thos Tegg Nº 111 Cheapside.

Rowlandson. Del

THE ANATOMIST.

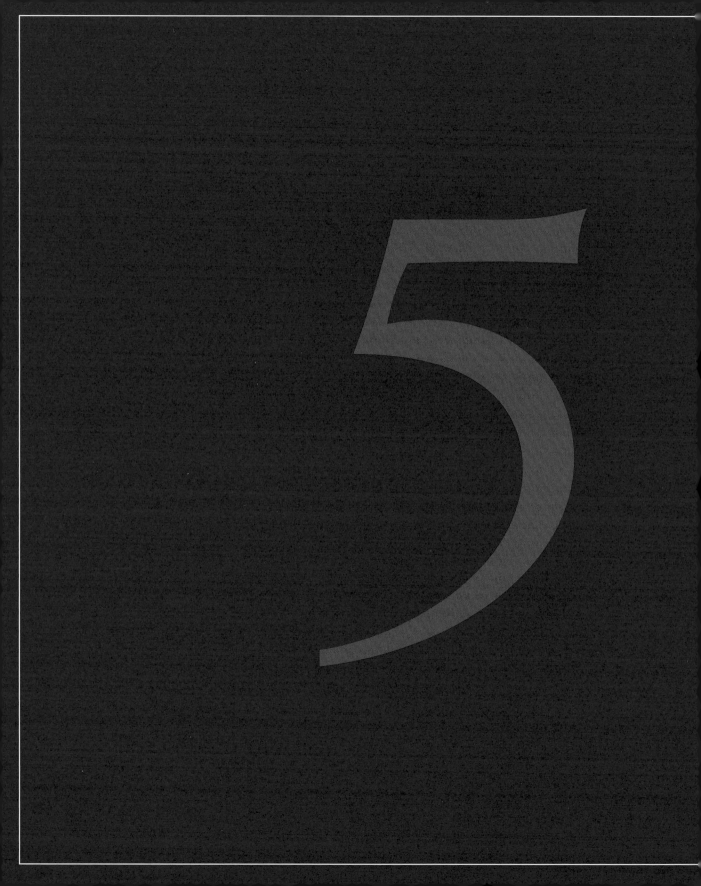

THE AGE OF ENLIGHTENMENT
1701–1800

After the breakthroughs of the sixteenth century and the goldrush of discoveries in the seventeenth, anatomy was in danger of becoming a commonplace pursuit in the eighteenth. In Britain, the century saw the status of surgeons elevated, a rapid but unregulated rise in the establishment of anatomy schools, and an increasing lay interest in public dissections. All of this contributed to a chronic shortage of cadavers, a problem which led to solutions by fair means and foul, by legal and illegal channels.

By the beginning of the eighteenth century, anatomy in England was dominated by the trade's guild, the Company of Barber-Surgeons. Surgeons and barbers first became associated on the battlefield, where barbers, possessing sharp razors and a degree of hand-eye coordination, were as likely to be asked to conduct an amputation as to cut hair. Physicians, with their academic medical training, considered themselves superior to barber-surgeons, who (except in Italy) were taught merely in apprenticeships. To improve their skills with a knife, surgeons learned to cut hair and shave faces before they were taught anatomy. Physicians generally disassociated themselves from all forms of surgery – not least because survival rates from operations were very low. Traditionally physicians could use the prefix 'doctor', but surgeons were only addressed as 'mister'.

The skill of barber-surgeons increased, partly from the rise in anatomical knowledge and partly from the new injuries of war – wounds were no longer caused by the relatively simple weapons of blade and arrow but by the blunt force of musket and cannon balls. It was in war that surgeons gained the bulk of their experience, both as apprentices and as qualified practitioners. The Company of Barber-Surgeons, which had a monopoly of dissections, was allowed to perform only ten a year at the start of the eighteenth century, up from a mere four a hundred years earlier.

1 William Cheselden

The Company forbade its members from undertaking unauthorised autopsies; and, although permission to dissect must be sought, it was never granted, and anyone who went ahead was censured and fined £10. Its monopoly was in any case often ignored by anatomists seeking to further their knowledge or income. One young Englishman, William Cheselden, openly challenged the authority of the Company (of which he was a member) by offering a program of thirty-five lectures in human anatomy in his London home over the winter of 1713/14. Cheselden (1688–1752) studied under the plagiarist-anatomist William Cowper. He complained that the Company's monopolistic practices were restricting the advancement of anatomy out of fear that bright young members such as he were outstripping its elderly ruling members.

His lectures were intended not only to challenge the Company but to promote his new book, *The Anatomy of the Humane Body*, a handbook for students which achieved great popularity, largely because it was written in English and not Latin. From its publication in 1713 it went through fifteen English editions and one German one. By 1806 three editions had been printed in the young United States. The first edition contained twenty-seven images (rising to forty by the sixth) whose accuracy was improved by the use of a camera obscura during their preparation.

This was a modern book, technologically advanced and readable in one's own language. *The Anatomy of the Humane Body* placed the emphasis on practical surgery with

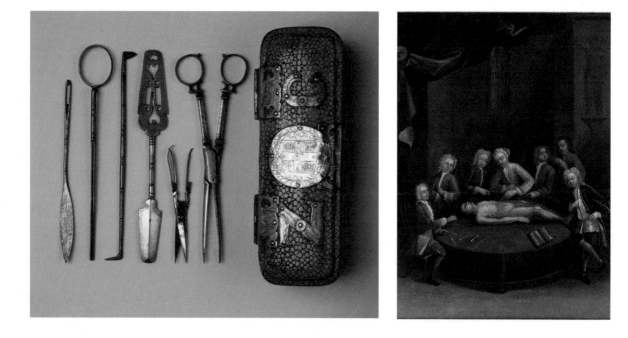

the inclusion of case studies and surgical techniques. Cheselden was himself an innovative surgeon who developed new procedures for cataracts of the eye and the removal of gallstones – the latter took minutes instead of hours, and reduced the mortality of such an operation to less than 10 per cent.

Cheselden's *Humane Body* was his most successful publication, but in 1733 he wrote a more significant work of anatomy, *Osteographia, or The Anatomy of Bones*. It was the first full account of the human skeleton, a work of art and scholarship. It contained eighty-eight illustrations, engraved by Gerard Vandergucht and Jacob Schijnvoet. Vandergucht was the London-born son of a Flemish engraver, from whom he learned his craft; besides his contribution to Cheselden's book he was an ardent campaigner for artists' royalties to be extended to prints, not just original works. Fifty-six of his plates for *Osteographia* were reproduced twice in the book: once with reference letters linking to text on the back of each one, and once without them, so that they could be appreciated as images in their own right. Schijnvoet, a Dutchman who worked on both sides of the English Channel, contributed beautifully delicate illustrations of both human and animal skeletal anatomy.

William Cheselden was the finest surgeon in England during his life, and his *Anatomy of the Humane Body* had a lasting impact on anatomy, not only at home but around the world. It placed Britain at the forefront of anatomical advances for the next hundred years or so. Its American editions spread his influence to the New World, and – revised and updated by the medical missionary Benjamin Hobson in the early nineteenth century – it played a part in transforming Chinese and Japanese medical practice.

His criticisms of the Company of Barber-Surgeons bore fruit in 1745 when a new company was established by royal decree, the Company of Surgeons, later to become the

ABOVE LEFT

An English surgeon's tool kit (1650s)

The case is made of silver-mounted sharkskin and carries the arms of the Barber-Surgeons' Company

ABOVE RIGHT

William Cheselden Giving an Anatomical Demonstration (c.1730)

This oil painting is attributed to Charles Phillips (1703–47), an English painter of society portraits.

*The Anatomy of the
Humane Body* (1713)

The foetal heart, etched for
William Cheselden's textbook
by Gerard Vandergucht
(1696–1776), an English artist
of Flemish descent.

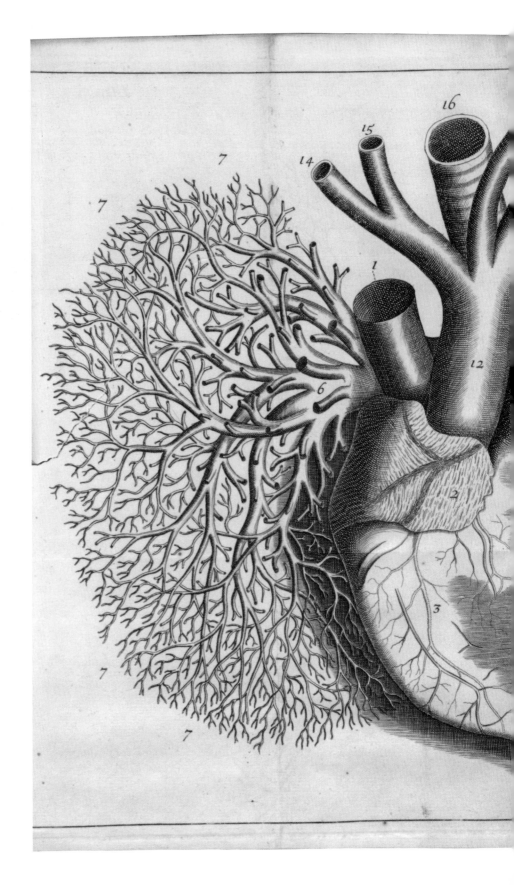

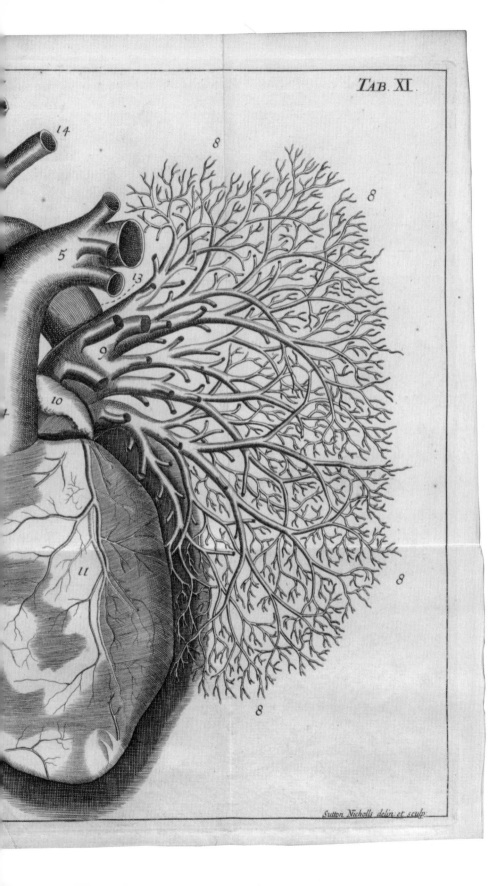

Sutton Nicholls delin: et sculp.

Osteographia (1733)

Cheselden's anatomy of the bones is a work of art and scholarship. This image shows the rib cage, spine and pelvis from the rear.

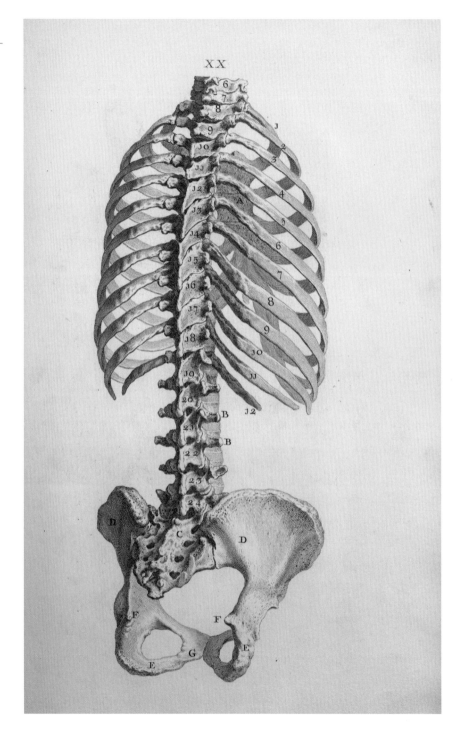

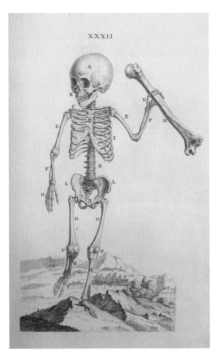

XXXII

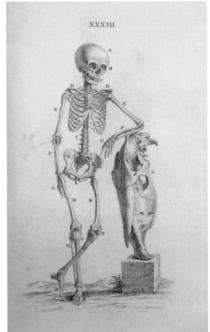

XXXIII

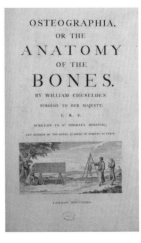

OSTEOGRAPHIA,
OR THE
ANATOMY
OF THE
BONES.
BY WILLIAM CHESELDEN
SURGEON TO HER MAJESTY:
F. R. S.
SURGEON TO ST THOMAS'S HOSPITAL,
AND MEMBER OF THE ROYAL ACADEMY OF SURGERY AT PARIS.

LONDON MDCCXXXIII.

Osteographia (1733)

Above left: The skeleton of
an eighteen-month-old child
carries an adult femur for
comparison. Above centre: The
skeleton of a nine-year-old boy
leaning on an animal skull.
Above right: The title page of
the first full account of the
skeleton. Far left: The skull in
horizontal and vertical sections.

LEFT

Samuel Wood (1737)

Samuel Wood's right arm was
torn off at the shoulder by a
windmill on 15 August 1737.
He survived and underwent
an operation at St Thomas'
Hospital by Mr Ferne, a
surgeon. At least two different
engravings of this medical
marvel were produced for
public sale.

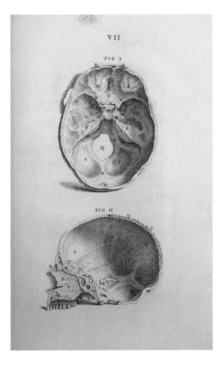

VII

FIG I

FIG II

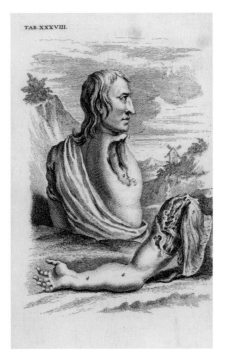

TAB. XXXVIII.

Royal College of Surgeons. The Worshipful Company of Barbers continued to occupy the Barber-Surgeons' Hall, on a site which had been chosen for its proximity to Newgate Prison, from which corpses often became available for dissection. Its anatomy theatre (until its demolition in 1784) was the only part of the original building to survive the Great Fire of London.

2 William and John Hunter, and William Smellie

The secession of the surgeons marked their transition from craft practice to professionalism, and at last broke the Barber-Surgeons' monopoly. In 1746, a Scottish anatomist called William Hunter offered an anatomy course with the novel attraction of hands-on experience of dissection. He had seen this for himself when he studied anatomy in Paris, and it seemed obvious to him that young surgeons would be less likely to kill the living if they had first practiced on the dead.

Hunter (1718–83) was the first of a new wave of anatomy teachers enabled by the surgeons' breakaway. He eventually built his own anatomy theatre in London where many of the next generation of anatomists were taught their trade. One of Hunter's early publications was a 1743 treatise on the joints, *On the Structure and Diseases of Articulating Cartilages*. He became Queen Caroline's obstetrician in 1764 and his greatest contribution to anatomy was *Anatomia uteri humani gravidi tabulis illustrata* (*The Anatomy of the Human Gravid Uterus Exhibited in Figures*), written in 1774, with plates of the physiology of pregnancy engraved by another Dutchman, Jan van Rymsdyk.

Hunter had studied obstetrics under William Smellie (1697–1763), a fellow Scot and one of the first male midwives in an understandably female-dominated profession. It's all the more remarkable that Smellie was self-taught and gained a degree from the University of Glasgow only after he had been teaching the subject successfully in London for many years. Smellie brought a scientific mind to the subject. He devised a manikin to help his students understand the birthing process and offered free midwifery to clients on condition that they allow his students to observe. Smellie designed a less invasive form of obstetrical forceps, and by the time he retired to Scotland in 1759 he had delivered over a thousand babies and taught nearly 300 courses. In retirement he completed his life's work: *A Treatise on the Theory and Practice of Midwifery*. Although some resented the involvement of a man in the intimate moments of birth, no one could deny the value of his experience. He published separately a collection of his own obstetrical drawings, *A Sett of Anatomical Tables* (1754), which were ground-breaking in their detail.

Smellie passed his knowledge on to around 900 pupils. William Hunter's courses were also popular, and enrolment for them rose from twenty in 1748 to 100 by 1756. Under the rules of the Company of Surgeons a license to practice was only granted after an applicant had attended two courses of anatomy. Other surgeons quickly saw the opportunity to increase their income and many more schools were established in the second half of the century. The lectures of Cheselden, Hunter and others created a sellers' market in the provision of bodies for dissection. There were not enough legally available corpses, so gangs of criminals, known euphemistically to anatomists as resurrectionists for their practice of raising the dead, took to exhuming recently buried bodies from graveyards and selling them to anatomy schools.

BELOW
William Hunter (1718–83)

A portrait by the Scottish artist Allan Ramsay (1713–84).

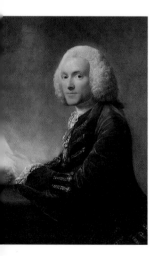

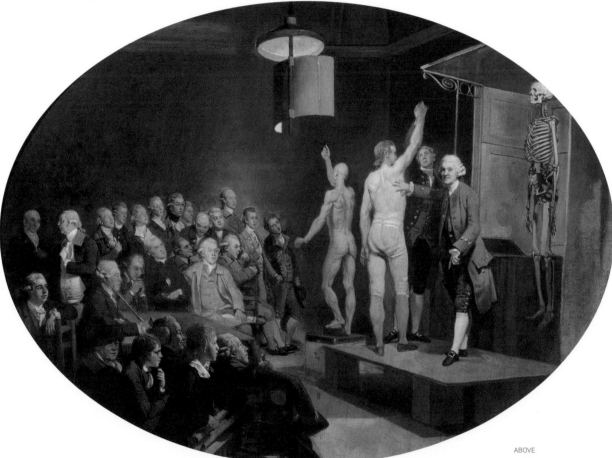

**William Hunter giving an
anatomy demonstration**

A painting by Johann Zoffany
(1733–1810) shows Hunter
using a living model and an
écorché statue. Behind him is
a very tall skeleton, possibly
that of Charles Byrne, the Irish
Giant, which was acquired by
Hunter's brother John.

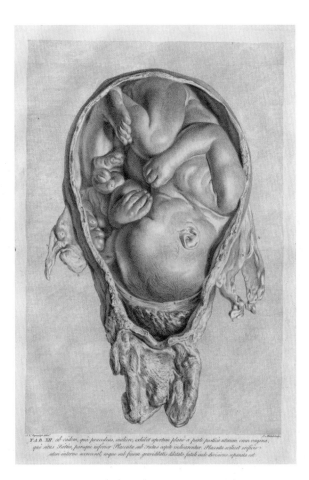

*Anatomia uteri
humani gravidi
tabulis illustrata* (1774)

Right: A foetus in utero, from
William Hunter's study of
the physiology of pregnancy.
Opposite: Hunter's book
contains meticulous drawings
from every stage of dissection.

In an attempt to remedy this unsavoury state of affairs the British government passed
the Murder Act in 1752. This ruled that executed murderers would be further punished
by being dissected after their death. It became the custom to make a token 'official'
incision at the place of execution before the body was then removed to one of the medical
schools for more detailed invasion. The aim of the Act was twofold: to discourage murder
by playing on the general public's continuing revulsion of dissection, while at the same
time providing more cadavers for anatomists.

The Act's success in one of those aims, however, would inevitably be its undoing in
the other. And so it transpired: murder was indeed discouraged, and the number of
hangings in England went down during the eighteenth century, despite a later increase in
the number of crimes punishable by death; so there were fewer legally dissectible cadavers
than ever. The same crisis of supply was affecting many European countries, which passed
laws allowing the use of the bodies of paupers, psychiatric patients and prisoners who had
died naturally. Britain, however, only passed such legislation in the early nineteenth
century, and in the eighteenth business boomed for graverobbers and even murderers

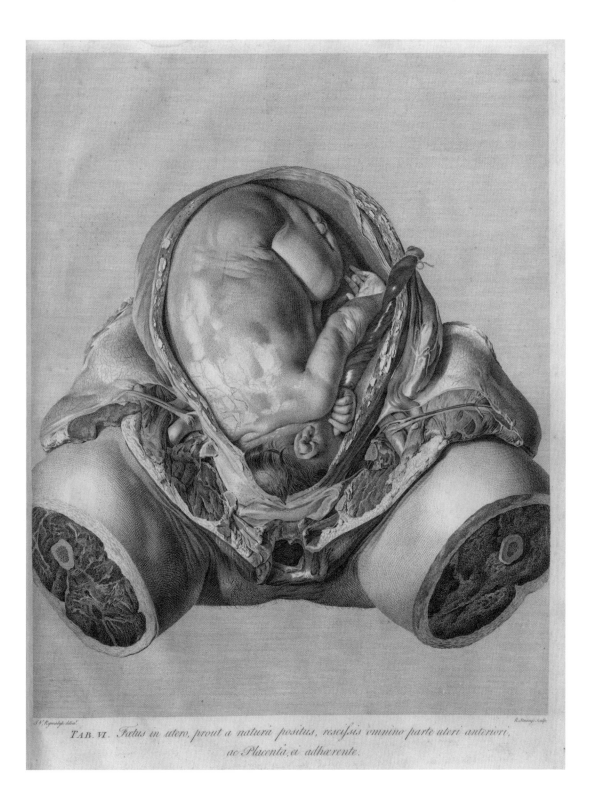

TAB. VI. *Fœtus in utero, prout a naturâ positus, rescissis omnino parte uteri anteriori, ac Placentâ ei adhærente.*

The Theory and Practice of Midwifery (1764)

William Hunter's tutor William Smellie had attended over a thousand births by the time he completed his textbook on midwifery. Below left: The use of forceps in delivery. Below right: A baby with its umbilical cord wrapped around its neck and arm. Opposite: Twins in the womb.

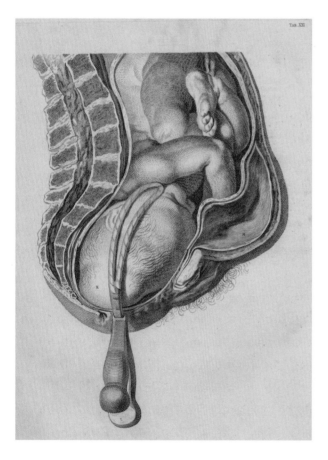

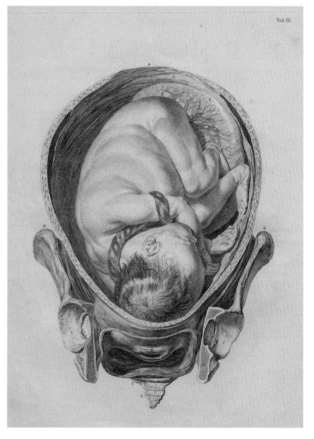

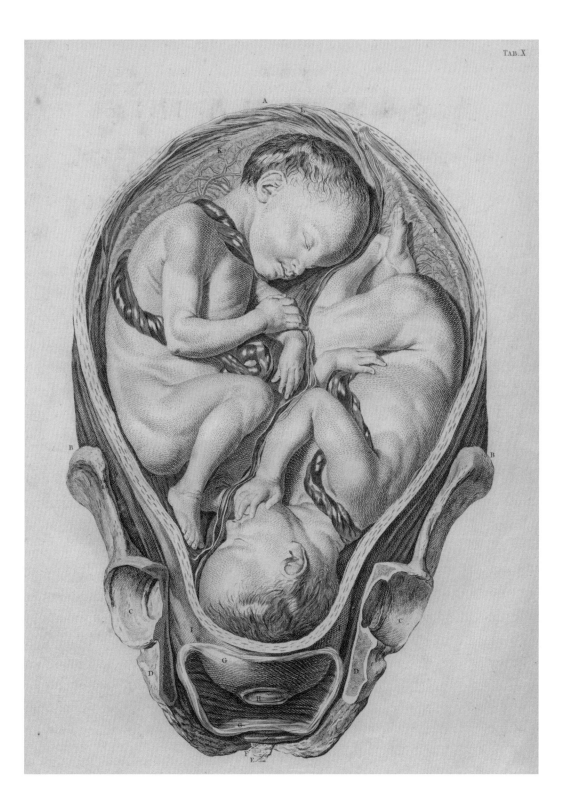

TAB. X

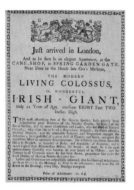

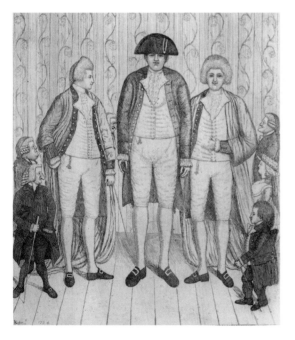

who killed their victims purely in order to sell them to anatomy schools. Communities responded by appointing watchmen to guard cemeteries and by providing iron body-safes in which the deceased would be kept until the body had passed its usefulness to dissectors and could safely be buried.

In the twenty-first century, one researcher accused William Hunter (without, it must be said, much evidence) of murdering the pregnant women whose conditions he studied in *The Anatomy of the Human Gravid Uterus*. It is probably untrue; but there is evidence that his younger brother John Hunter, also a gifted anatomist, did procure cadavers on the black market. John (1728–93) learned anatomy as his brother's assistant during dissections and studied under William Cheselden. He was interested in inflammation, which he recognised as a reaction of the body, not a cause of illness. Having worked as an army surgeon for several years, he was regarded as an expert on venereal diseases, about which he wrote a treatise in 1786. He was wrong in believing that gonorrhoea and syphilis were aspects of the same infection; but he carried out the first recorded human artificial insemination, for the wife of a linen draper.

John Hunter was a compulsive collector of specimens. He preserved the organs and skeletons of humans and animals; at his death he had some 14,000 examples, which today form part of the Hunterian Museum in London, named in his honour. With or without William's knowledge he may well have acquired bodies for his brother's demonstrations and certainly did for his own anatomy school, established in 1764 after he left the army.

His most notorious cadaver was that of Charles Byrne, 2.31m (7ft 7in) tall and popularly known as the Irish Giant in freak shows around the country. Byrne declined Hunter's ghoulish request to have his body after his death and, suspecting that his refusal would not be enough, asked friends to bury him at sea. He was thwarted, however, when Hunter paid a hearse driver £500 to replace the body with rocks during an overnight stop on its journey to the coast. In 1787 Hunter displayed Byrne's unusual skeleton in his museum. It is, to this day, in the collection of the Hunterian Museum, where it formed a centrepiece in a glass case for the next 200 years. For anatomists with a fiction section in their libraries, the author Hilary Mantel has written an imagined account of the lives of Charles Byrne and John Hunter called *The Giant, O'Brien* (1998), which juxtaposes an Irish culture of song and legend with the emerging, matter-of-fact Scientific Age.

There is a distinct clash between the distaste for dissection still felt in the eighteenth century by the general public and the enthusiasm for anatomy among the educated classes. Sons of the wealthy liberal elite were expected to have at least a passing knowledge of anatomy and other sciences, even if they had no intention of pursuing them professionally; and many of the new anatomy schools catered for this lay interest. But the antipathy of the public towards this cold-hearted scientific use of the human frame, home of the soul, was the moral opposite of the desperate need for bodies to advance the science.

The lack of corpses, and popular opposition to the science, both acted to slow the pace of discovery in the eighteenth century. It is significant that many of the seventeenth-century texts still in print in the eighteenth century added no updated information from one edition to the next. The works of William Cheselden are a good example. The focus was on the application of existing anatomical knowledge to the practices of surgery and physiology, not on new discoveries of anatomical detail. This was a century largely of consolidation, and its publications are often to be enjoyed for the quality of their illustrations as for the quantity of their anatomical innovations.

3 Bernhard Siegfried Albinus

Tabulae sceleti et musculorum corporis humani (*Diagrams of the Skeleton and Muscles of the Human Body*) by Bernhard Siegfried Albinus is a case in point. When it was published in 1747 it covered the same ground that Cheselden's *Osteographia* had only fourteen years earlier. But it is a beautiful book. Albinus (1697–1770) unexpectedly drew criticism for the light-heartedness of its illustrations, by the artist and engraver Jan Wandelaar of the northern Netherlands.

Wandelaar and Albinus devised a system of net squares through which to view the skeletal subjects of the images in order to achieve greater accuracy. Albinus must, however, have given Wandelaar a free hand in designing the backgrounds of the anatomical figures. The frontal view of a full-length skeleton is thrown into relief by a billowing cloak held behind it by a flying cherub. It looks as if the cherub has dramatically whipped off the cloth (or perhaps the skin) to reveal the bones in all their glory. Even more startling are two other images of partially muscled skeletons (known technically as 'fourth order' for the level of musculature on show). In the background of these front and rear views, a disinterested rhinoceros stands, gazing into the distance. The rhinoceros in question was Clara, the first of her species to arrive in Europe. Wandelaar's sensational engravings, the first anatomically correct images of a rhinoceros, were released five years before *Tabulae sceleti* was completed as an advertisement of the book's accuracy.

Albinus is the Latin form of the family's German surname Weiss. Bernhard Siegfried Albinus was a fine anatomist and the son of another – his father Bernhard Albinus brought the family to Holland from their native Germany in order to take up the chair of anatomy at the University of Leiden. Albinus junior began to study medicine there at the age of twelve, when his teachers were Hermann Boerhaave and Nicolaas Bidloo. In time, he followed his father in the professorship, and his brother – Frederick Bernhard Albinus – followed him. Although he is not credited with any great discoveries or innovation, Bernhard Siegfried Albinus was a prolific author. He wrote several treatises on bones and muscles, on blood circulation and on skin pigmentation. With his former teacher, Boerhaave, he also edited the works of his illustrious predecessors Vesalius and Harvey.

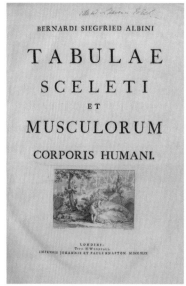

Tabulae sceleti et musculorum corporis humani (1747)

A skeleton displaying fourth order musculature is as unaware of Clara the rhinoceros as she is of it. Clara, something of a celebrity, was the first of her species to arrive in Europe.

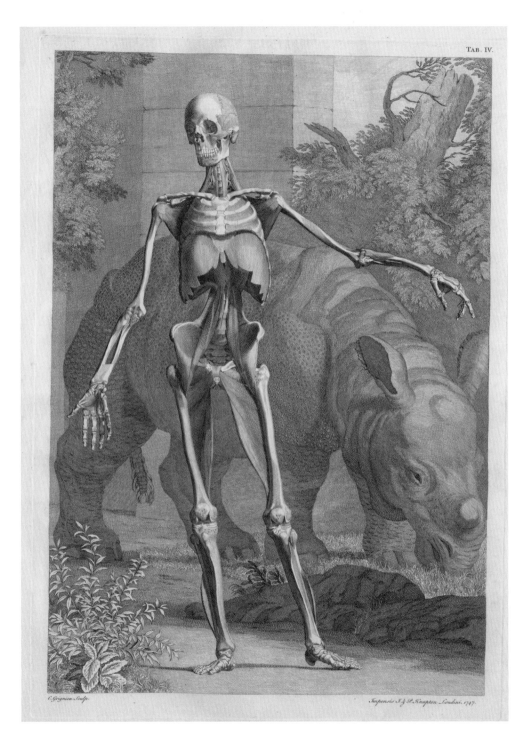

TAB. IV.

C. Grignion Sculp.

Impensis I. & P. Knapton Londini. 1747.

4 Jacques-François-Marie Duverney and Jacques Fabien Gautier d'Agoty

Britain and the Netherlands were in the ascendency in the eighteenth century. But France and Italy continued to exert their influence. William Hunter advertised his lectures as being 'in the same manner as at Paris'. One family dominated the Parisian scene in the first half of the eighteenth century, if only by weight of numbers. Three brothers – Joseph-Guichard Duverney, Pierre Duverney and Jacques-François-Marie Duverney – were all practising anatomists, as was Joseph-Guichard's son Emmanuel-Maurice.

Anatomical interest resides chiefly in Jacques-François-Marie (1661–1748), the first man to describe the tensor tarsi muscle, which controls the tear ducts in the corner of the eye. Like many other discoverers, Jacques-François-Marie lost out to history, and the muscle is known today as Horner's muscle after the distinguished nineteenth-century Virginian anatomist, William Horner, who redescribed it in 1824.

Publishing interest focusses on books for which Jacques-François-Marie rarely gets the credit, but which are landmarks in the anatomist's library. Instead, his works are almost always listed under the name of their illustrator, Jacques Fabien Gautier d'Agoty. Gautier (1716–85) was a printer, engraver, painter and anatomist. He studied with the German artist Jakob Christoph Le Blon, who in 1708 had invented a colour-printing process based on the use of yellow, red and blue intaglio plates. He also devised a method of weaving tapestry using only black, white, yellow, red and blue thread. Le Blon had some initial success in England with his printing technique, but it didn't catch on and he returned to Paris to teach art to pupils such as Gautier and the Dutch engraver Jan L'Admiral.

L'Admiral refined Le Blon's method by adding a fourth, black plate and in 1737 printed an edition of one of Albinus's early works, which may have been the first full-colour book of anatomy. Gautier also added a black plate to Le Blon's three; and much to the outrage of Le Blon's family after his death, Gautier patented the process in his own name without acknowledging either Le Blon or L'Admiral.

Gautier wrote several books of anatomy, sharing dissection duties with Jacques-François-Marie Duverney and illustrating them with his own artwork. The first, in 1746, was a study of human musculature with twenty plates, *Myologie complette en couleur et grandeur naturelle: composée de l'essai et de la suite de l'essai d'anatomie en tableaux imprimés: ouvrage unique, utile et nécessaire aux etudians et amateurs de cette science* (*Complete Myology in Colour and Natural Size: Composed of the Essay and its Sequel on Anatomy in Printed Tables: Unique Work, Useful and Necessary for Students and Amateurs of this Science*). It was followed two years later by *Anatomie de la tête* (*Anatomy of the Head*), with eight plates, in whose extended title Duverney received an acknowledgement for his part in it.

Gautier's third book, published in 1752 after Duverney's death, addressed his absence. 'The loss of Mr Duverney is repaired by Mr Mertrud, who will continue the dissections.' That book, *Anatomie générale des viscères en situation: de grandeur et couleur naturelle, avec l'angeologie, et la nevrologie de chaque partie du corps humain* (*General Anatomy of the Viscera in Situation: of Natural Size and Colour, with the Angiology, and the Neurology of Each Part of the Human Body*), contained another eighteen plates and is considered Gautier's best work. For it, he conducted all but three of the dissections himself.

RIGHT AND BELOW

Myologie complette en couleur et grandeur naturelle (1746)

Anatomy in full colour caused a sensation among the general public. Right: The title page. Below: The muscles of the neck, tongue and jaws.

FAR RIGHT

Anatomie générale des viscères en situation (1752)

The muscles of the limbs with a view of the abdominal cavity.

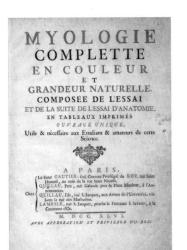

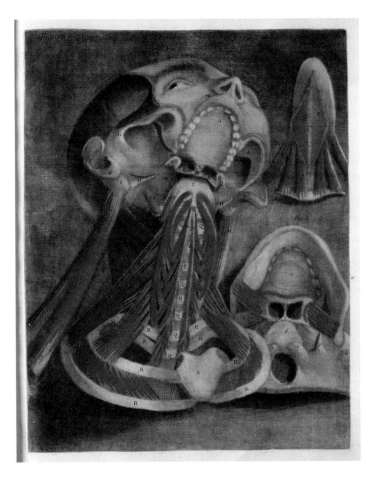

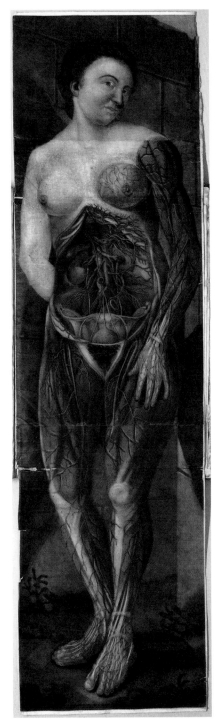

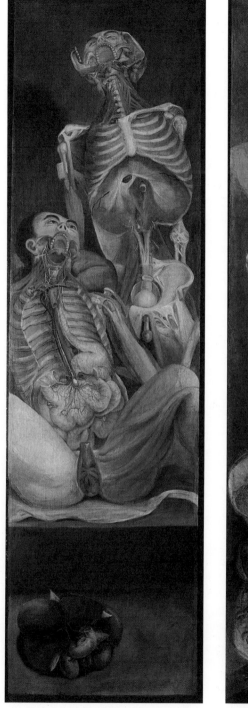

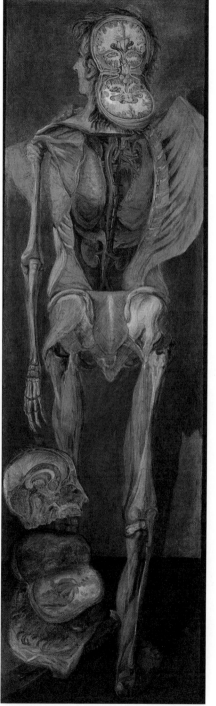

Anatomie générale des viscères en situation (1752)

Far left: A double portrait showing the digestive organs and the urinary system, with other viscera in the foreground. Left: Muscles and viscera from the rear, with the brain exposed and other sections of the brain at bottom left.

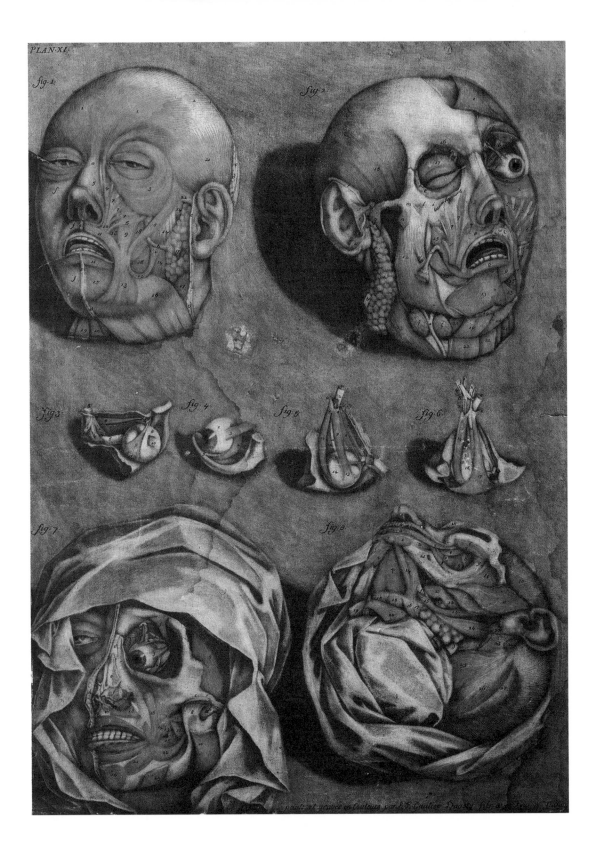

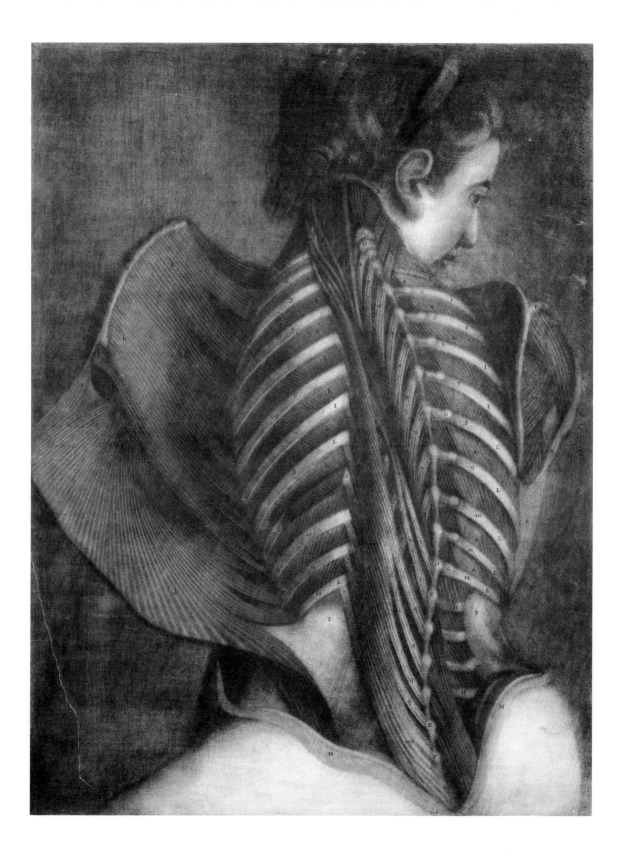

PREVIOUS PAGES

Myologie complette en couleur et grandeur naturelle (1746)

Left: Muscles of the face and eyes. Right: Partial dissection of a seated woman showing the bones and muscles of the back and shoulders.

BELOW

De aure humana tractatus (1735)

The title page of Antonio Maria Valsalva's monograph on the anatomy of the ear.

OPPOSITE

De aure humana tractatus (1735)

A view of the base of the skull, with the lower jaw removed, looking upward to the ears.

The colour illustrations must have been a sensation in their day and they combine anatomical images with an artistic flair for presentation. As a result, however, they look more like still life compositions than anatomy diagrams and lack the detail which would have been truly 'useful and necessary for students.' In retrospect, the German medical historian Johann Ludwig Choulant wrote in 1852, 'His anatomical illustrations, while they may perhaps be fascinating to the layman, impress the critical observer with their arrogance and charlatanery and do not recommend themselves to the student of anatomy either for their faithfulness or their technique.' Gautier may be better remembered for *Observations sur l'histoire naturelle* (*Natural History Observations*), one of the earliest French scientific journals, which he launched in 1752 and which ran until the last year of the century.

Duverney did publish work under his own name as well as under Gautier's, including: *Traité de l'organe de l'ouïe, contenant la structure, les usages et les maladies de toutes les parties de l'oreille* (*Treatise on the Organ of Hearing, Containing the Structure, Uses and Diseases of all Parts of the Ear*) in 1731, with sixteen unsigned but detailed black and white plates, probably based on Duverney's own drawings; and, posthumously in 1749, *L'art de disséquer méthodiquement les muscles du corps humain, mis à la portée des commençans* (*The Art of Methodically Dissecting the Muscles of the Human Body, Made Accessible to Beginners*).

5 Giovanni Battista Morgagni, Antonio Maria Valsalva and Théophile Bonet

At the University of Padua, the professor of anatomy for most of the eighteenth century was Giovanni Battista Morgagni, who held the post for fifty-six years from 1712 to his death in 1771. He trained at Padua's rival Bologna, where he acted as prosector to a student of Marcello Malpighi, Antonio Maria Valsalva. Valsalva occupied the position of demonstrator of anatomy at the University of Bologna, and Morgagni contributed to Valsalva's important

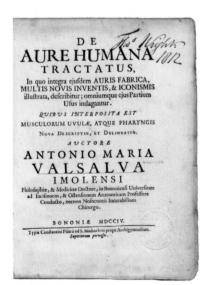

1735 work *De aure humana tractatus* (*A Treatise on the Human Ear*), a study of aural anatomy and disease. Valsalva is commemorated today in the Valsalva device, fitted in spacesuits to allow astronauts to equalise the pressure in their ears without using their hands to block their nose (that more usual hands-on method being known as the Valsalva manoeuvre).

As a tutor, Morgagni (1682–1771) discouraged medical speculation and insisted that his students use detailed observation and logic to reach diagnoses. He had a reputation as a brilliant anatomist; but for most of his tenure at Padua he concentrated on teaching, publishing only a few medical papers from 1706–19 under the title *Adversaria anatomica* (*Anatomical Adversaries*) on subjects such as gallstones, varicose veins and medico-legal dilemmas.

Then, all at once, at the age of seventy-nine, he published his life's work in *De sedibus et causis morborum per anatomen indagatis* (*Of the Seats and Causes of Diseases Investigated through Anatomy*). It was a huge book – twenty years in the writing, with five sections in two substantial volumes – and it not only encapsulated the knowledge of a lifetime but almost single-handedly launched the science of anatomical pathology.

TAB. IV.

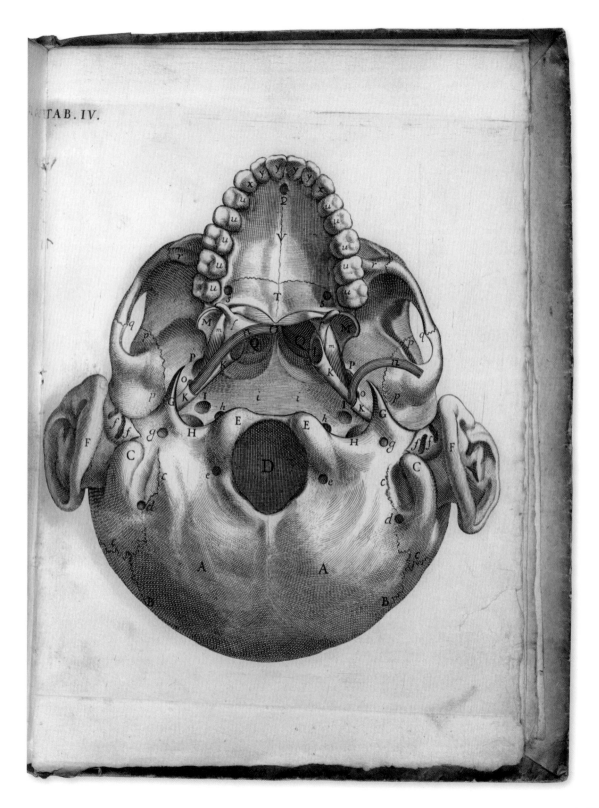

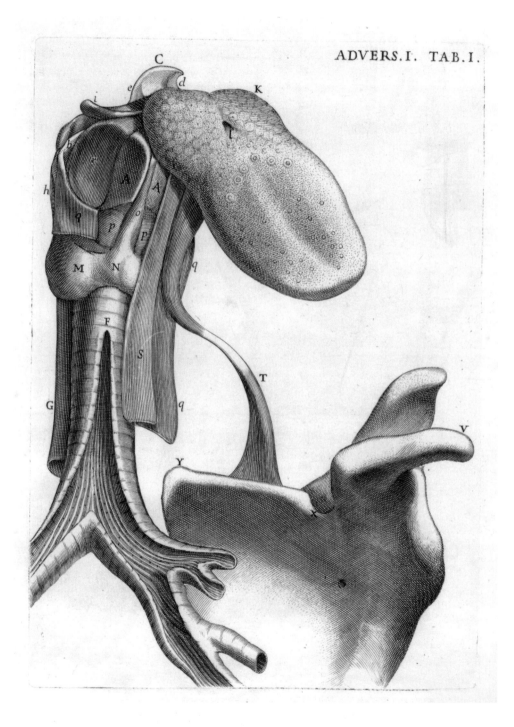

While centuries of dissection had produced a fairly complete image of normal human anatomy, few had studied the anatomy of organs which had become diseased. William Harvey had noted in the seventeenth century that 'there is more to be learned from the dissection of one person who had died of tuberculosis or other chronic malady than from the bodies of ten persons who had been hanged [while in otherwise good physical health].' In *De sedibus* Morgagni referred to the only other significant work in the field, *Sepulchretum: sive anatomia practica ex cadaveribus morbo denatis* (*The Cemetery, or Anatomy Practiced from Corpses Dead of Disease*), written by the Swiss physician Théophile Bonet in 1679.

Morgagni considered Bonet's to be a derivative work, drawing on other men's works and focussing on morbidly fascinating and extreme examples of diseased organs. Others admire him for having drawn together all the pathological knowledge of others to date. If Bonet (1620–89) lacked scientific rigour, Morgagni more than made up for it. He was a meticulous record keeper and in the book he refers to his contemporary observations of 646 dissections, most of them conducted by him.

De sedibus takes the form of seventy letters which Morgagni wrote to a friend who had encouraged him to commit his knowledge to paper. The format makes it difficult to navigate as a reference work, but is precious as an insight into a pioneer's processes. The book was immediately successful: it was reprinted four times in its first three years, and within ten years it had been translated into French, German and English.

6 Anatomy in Japan

The history of anatomy is principally a European one. In the Far East, medicine remained a largely non-invasive discipline. For example, Japan's medical system, *kanpō*, was based on Chinese knowledge first imported in the sixth century. *Kanpō* included acupuncture, moxibustion, herbology and food therapy. Japan had been a closed society since 1639, trading only with China and some outposts of the Dutch East Indian empire, and only via the port of Nagasaki. Japanese physicians were, however, as curious as European ones; and showed a tentative interest in anatomy from the fourteenth century onwards.

The first scientific dissections in Japan did not take place until the eighteenth century, but earlier publications showed a simple grasp of the major organs. Some dissection of executed criminals did take place before then, and a fifty-volume book, *Tonisho* (*Book of the Simple Physician*) written in 1304 by the priest-physician Kajiwara Shōzen (1266–1337), included one volume on rudimentary anatomy, illustrated with diagrammatic woodcuts.

Jesuit missionaries brought some expertise in European surgery with them in the sixteenth century, but they were regarded as 'southern barbarians' by the local populations. After 1639, those dealing with Dutch traders at Nagasaki might have had some experience of their medical practices, which was known as *komogeka* (red-haired surgery) or *orandageka* (Holland surgery). One interpreter, Ryoi Motoki (1628–97), is known to have completed a rough translation of a Dutch edition of Johan Remmelin's *A Mirror of the Microcosm* around 1680, although it wasn't published until 1772.

Tōyō Yamawaki (1705–62) was the first Japanese physician to challenge some of the traditional beliefs of *kanpō*. In 1754 he was given permission to dissect the body of a

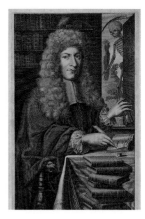

Adversaria anatomica omnia (1723)

Opposite: The muscles of the tongue and larynx. Top: A portrait of the author, Giovanni Battista Morgagni, who single-handedly launched the science of anatomical pathology. Above: The title page of a compilation of Morgagni's medical papers.

criminal who had been beheaded. He wrote *Zoshi* (*Notes on the Viscera*) over the next five years, noting the differences between those traditional ideas and his own observations, and furthermore the agreement between his observations and those contained in an unidentified European book of anatomy, possibly by the German anatomist Johann Vesling (1598–1649), to which he had access.

Zoshi aroused condemnation from traditionalists, but also rallied support from physicians of a more scientific mind. It opened a Japanese window onto contemporary European anatomy. In its wake, two books published in the space of two years showed just how willing and quick Japanese physicians were to learn from European advances.

In 1771 another dissection was allowed, this time of a female criminal. Three men among the audience had each brought along the same Dutch anatomy book, *Ontleedkundige tafelen* (*Anatomical Tables*), written by Johann Adam Kulmus and published in Amsterdam in 1734. Like Tōyō Yamawaki, they were struck by the accuracy of the book, and agreed that they should make a Japanese translation of it. It was an ambitious goal, not least because none of them knew more than a handful of Dutch words. Even if they did, there simply weren't the words in Japanese for the anatomical terms with which they were confronted.

Meanwhile in Kyoto, Kawaguchi Shinnin (1736–1811) rushed into print in 1772 with his own anatomy, *Kaishi hen* (*Analysis of Cadavers*), illustrated with woodcuts by the artist Aoki Shukuya (d. 1802). The images have a beautiful simplicity, uncluttered by excessive detail or labels, with a tendency to resort to pattern or symmetry where none exists, for example, in the neat coils of the intestines. It is a landmark publication in the Japanese history of anatomy, printed at the very dawn of the country's explorations of it.

The three worthy gentlemen from the anatomy demonstration set about learning Dutch, not only a foreign language but one written in an unfamiliar alphabet. One of them, Ryotaku Maeno (1723–1803), studied it with the interpreters of Nagasaki, then wrote a small booklet on the Dutch language to help his colleagues. Gempaku Sugita (1733–1817), with worse Dutch but greater enthusiasm for the project, became the lead author. Junnan Nakagawa (1739–86), the third of the original trio, was joined by Hoshu Katsuragawa (1751–1809). Over three and a half years they laboured painstakingly over each word, inventing a new Japanese anatomical lexicon as they went.

In 1774 they published Kulmus's book in Japanese as *Kaitai s hinsho* (*A New Book of Anatomy*). They used illustrations from many sources, not just Kulmus's. Some were from Juan Valverde's 1552 work *History of the Composition of the Human Body*, which Valverde had in turn 'borrowed' from Vesalius's *De fabrica*. Some first appeared in Govert Bidloo's 1685 *Anatomy of the Human Body*. The contrast with *Kaishi hen*, published only two years earlier, is stark. Where Kawaguchi Shinnin's images hark back to those of Shozen Kajiwara 400 years earlier, the Kulmus translation has all the realism and accurate detail of the eighteenth century. Although it was – strictly speaking – a Dutch work, its arrival in Japan, in Japanese, was enormously significant. Japan's policy of isolation continued until 1869, but western anatomy was one of the first sciences to break through the cordon, contributing to the general opening-up of Japan to European ideas in the later nineteenth century.

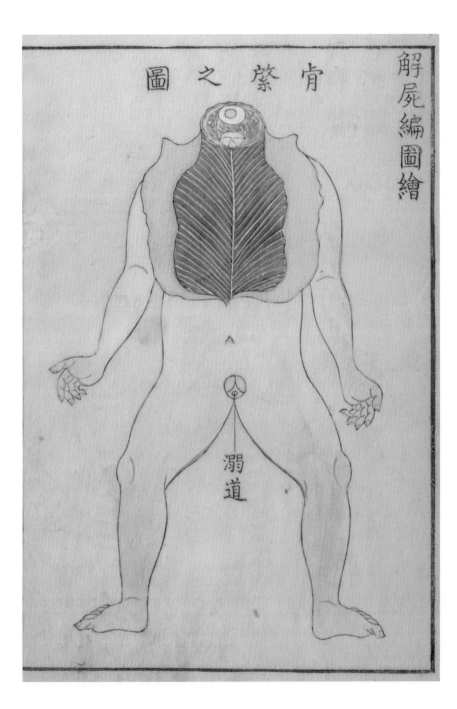

解屍編圖繪

宵綮之圖

溺道

LEFT

Kaishi hen (1772)

A woodcut by Aoki Shukuya
of a decapitated, partially
dissected figure, from the first
modern Japanese anatomy,
written by Kawaguchi Shinnin
(1736–1811).

The top of a head, with part of the skull removed, and a detail of the brain.

The title page of the Japanese translation of Johann Adam Kulmus's *Ontleedkundige tafelen* (1734) uses a very European architectural template.

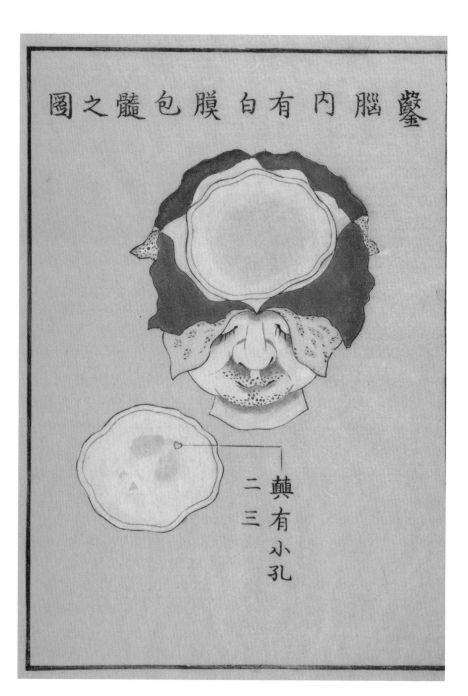

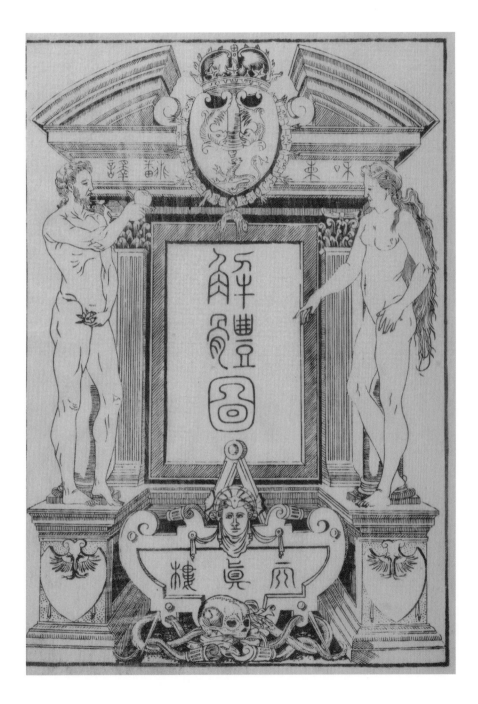

Kaitai shinsho (1774)

A sheet of images drawn
from various Asian and
European sources, showing the
diaphragm, the upper skeleton
and the viscera in male and
female cadavers. The flayed
torso, suspended by a rope,
is borrowed from Vesalius
(see page 104).

OPPOSITE

Kaitai shinsho (1774)

A man's head with the skull
exposed, and a hair follicle in
microscopic detail.

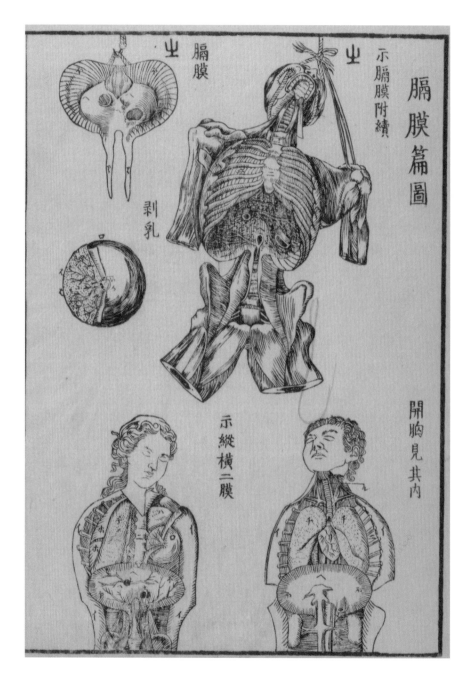

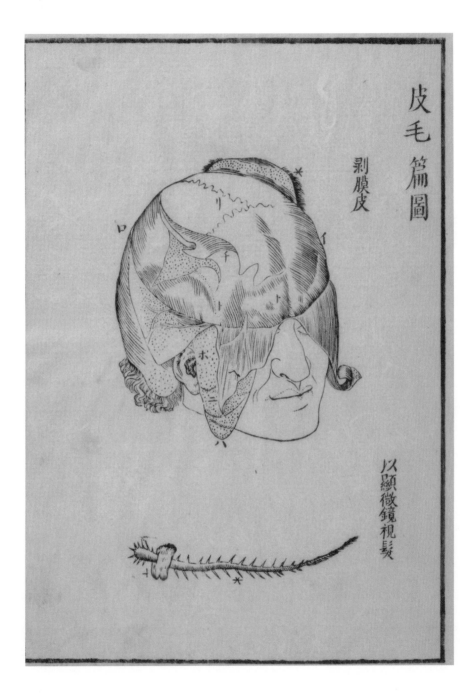

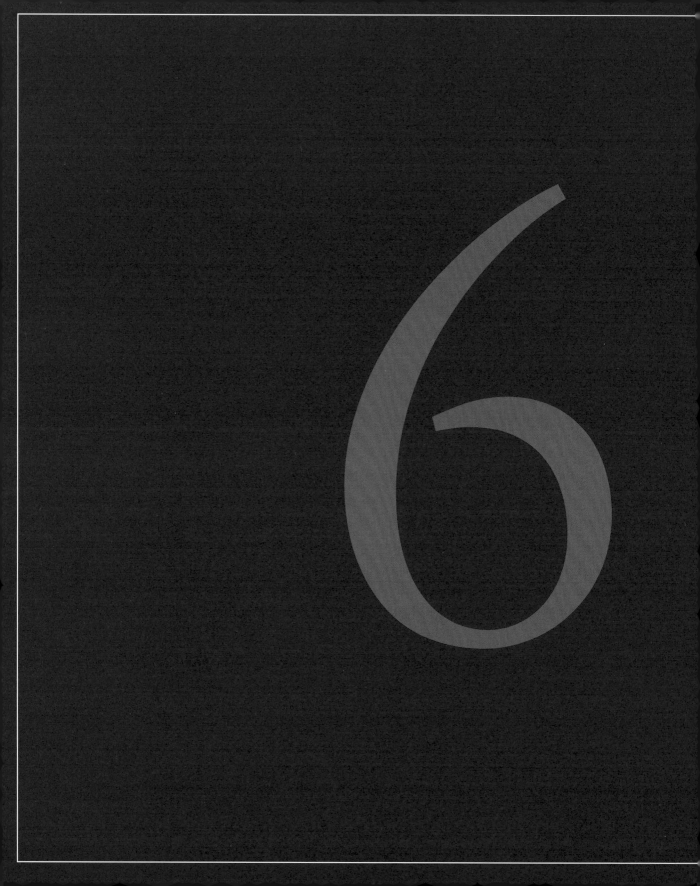

THE AGE OF INVENTION

1801–1900

After the consolidation of the accumulated knowledge of human anatomy in the eighteenth century, the nineteenth saw moves to codify it and protect it. Professional bodies and governments began to regulate training, but the public – with good reason – remained suspicious of the practice of dissection.

1 Hanaoka Seishū

Japan, having belatedly become aware of European approaches to anatomy, was racing to catch up and, in some cases, overtake the west. Hanaoka Seishū (1760–1835) was the finest Japanese surgeon of his day. Born in Kyoto and trained in traditional herbal medicine, he studied anatomy through *rangaku*, as exposure to western knowledge was called (literally it means 'Dutch learning', because it was originally through trade with Holland that Japan was first exposed to such ideas).

Hanaoka was intrigued by the work of a Chinese surgeon of the second century CE. Hua Tuo (*c*.145–220) was reputed to have carried out operations using a potion called *mafeisan* (powder of boiled hemp) which rendered his patients unconscious and somehow paralysed the muscles to make incisions easier. Hua Tuo took his recipe to the grave, burning his manuscripts just before his death; but medical historians think it may have included lovage, mandragora, moonflower and various strains of angelica and aconitum.

Hanaoka set about trying to recreate the formula using his knowledge of medicinal herbs. It took almost twenty years, and his wife lost her sight after one experimental batch. In 1804, however, he performed a mastectomy on a sixty-year-old cancer patient who had first drunk a medicine he called *tsūsensan*. Its active ingredients, modern analysis shows, were scopolamine, hyoscyamine, atropine, aconitine and angelicotoxin. It took effect about four hours after consumption, and the patient remained unconscious for up to twenty-four hours. Hanaoka's mastectomy is the first recorded surgery under anaesthesia of the modern era, more than forty years before such a landmark in the west.

In Japan at the time, it was the practice not to publish books but to write manuscripts for students and other interested readers to copy. Hanaoka wrote prolifically, and in 1805 he described the procedures which he used in that first mastectomy, in a paper entitled *Nyuigan chiken-roku* (*Findings on Breast Cancer*). Some of his papers were not only copied but illustrated by others, and *Kishitsu geryō zukan* (*Surgical Casebook*) was a bound set of collected works produced posthumously in 1837, illustrated by Tangetsu Higuchi (1822–*c*.1890). In the fiction section of an anatomist's library, one may also find *Hanaoka Seishū no tsuma* (*The Doctor's Wife* in translations), a much-admired novel written in 1966 by Sawako Ariyoshi and based on Hanaoka's life.

Patients flocked to Hanaoka's door in his lifetime, and his house in Kinokawa is still preserved as a shrine to his memory. It was his misfortune to live at a time when Japan's border was

BELOW
Kishitsu geryō zukan (1837)

An illustration by Tangetsu Higuchi (1822–90) from Hanaoka Seishū's *Surgical Casebook* showing a tumour on a woman's back.

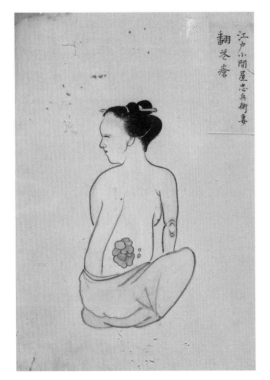

closed to the rest of the world, and his domestic fame never spread further afield. By the time the veil was lifted in 1854, nearly twenty years after his death, other techniques of anaesthesia had been invented in the west.

2 Leopoldo Marco Antonio Caldani, Antonio Scarpa and Domenico Cotugno

In Europe, the first decade of the new century was marked by several important publications. Three students of Giovanni Morgagni distinguished themselves in print. Leopoldo Caldani (1725–1813) trained in Bologna and at the University of Padua. At the latter he occupied the professorial chairs of both Theoretical Medicine and Anatomy, succeeding Morgagni. His fellow countryman, Alessandro Volta, invented the electrical battery in 1799, which for the first time gave scientists a stable supply with which to experiment; and Caldani experimented with electricity in the nervous system and on the functions of the spinal cord.

He retired in 1805, soon after the first publication of his best-known work, *Icones anatomicae* (*Anatomical Images*). It was printed in Venice, still a centre for anatomical artists, in stages over a period of thirteen years between 1801 and 1814, with help from Leopoldo's nephew Floriano Caldani. Its two volumes of illustrations, accompanied by

BELOW
Kishitsu geryō zukan (1837)

Left: Surgery to remove a tumour of the jawbone. Right: The fourth in a series of images illustrating breast cancer surgery.

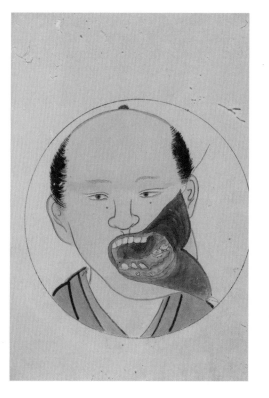

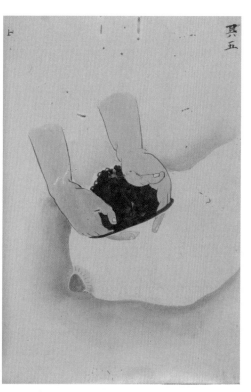

five of annotation, are considered among the finest of their kind. In their pages, graceful artistry combines with delicate detail in a way which would become obsolete over the course of the nineteenth century. Diagrams proved more functional and focussed as teaching aids; but one may mourn the lost elegance of these classical works.

Antonio Scarpa (1752–1832) studied under both Morgagni and Caldani at the University of Padua. Since the chair there was occupied, his career led him to professorships in Modena and Pavia; and his success at the latter prompted the university to build a new anatomy theatre, still known today as the Aula Scarpa – 'Scarpa Hall.' He was widely honoured for his work, both in Italy and abroad – elected a Fellow of Britain's Royal Society and a member of the Royal Swedish Academy of Sciences. When Napoleon Bonaparte became King of Italy in 1805, he visited Pavia and asked to meet Scarpa.

Scarpa died of an inflammation of the bladder brought on by the presence of a stone in his urinary system, and fittingly his body was dissected by his assistant Carlo Beolchin, who published a detailed account of the event. Less fittingly, in a misguided tribute to the great anatomist, his head was preserved and displayed in the university's Institute of Anatomy; and it is still on show in Pavia's University History Museum.

Scarpa was particularly interested in the brain and the organs of the senses, and in 1801 he published *Saggio di osservazioni e d'esperienze sulle principali malattie degli occhi* (*A Treatise on the Principal Diseases of the Eyes*), the first such work written in Italian. It followed his 1789 book (in Latin), *Anatomicae disquisitiones de auditu et olfactu* (*Anatomical Investigations of Hearing and Smell*). His best work was *Tabulae neurologicae* (*Neurological Records*) from 1794, in which, among other things, he gave the first complete description of the nerves of the heart. In it he also announced his discovery that the inner ear was filled with a fluid, subsequently known as Scarpa's fluid. He is also remembered in Scarpa's fascia, part of the lining of the abdomen, and in Scarpa's triangle, an area in the upper thigh.

Antonio Scarpa was known as a fierce man, ruthless with enemies and testing even with friends. When Napoleon visited him in Pavia, he had to be reinstated because he had been sacked for making unpopular political statements and refusing to take oaths. He never married but had many illegitimate sons for whom he used his influence to find lucrative positions. It is said that he locked the engraver of *Tabulae neurologicae* in his workshop until he had finished his task. He made many enemies who, after his death, launched attacks on his reputation. Some even vandalised memorials erected in his honour. There is no doubt, however, about his anatomical prowess.

In contrast, Domenico Cotugno (1736–1822) was a modest and cultured man and, in the context of the present book, much to be admired for his large library. From humble origins he learned his anatomy at Naples' Ospedale degli Incurabili (Hospital for Incurables), before travelling widely in pursuit of medical knowledge from Morgagni and others. He was Professor of Anatomy for thirty years in Naples where he impressed his students with a genuine spirit of medical enquiry aimed at the common good. To that end he wrote about sciatica and smallpox and, before Scarpa, about the aqueduct of the inner ear. Scarpa also acknowledged Cotugno's discovery of the nasopalatine nerve, which makes us sneeze. His collected works were published in four volumes as *Opera posthuma* (*Posthumous Works*) in 1830.

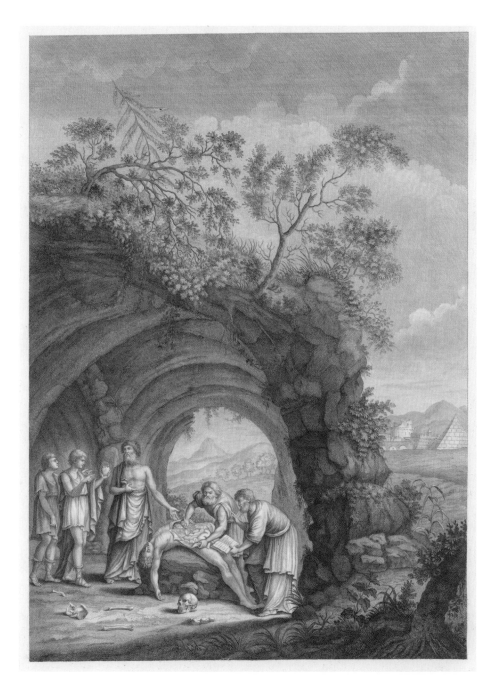

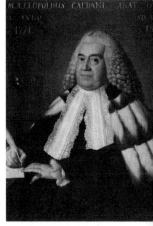

Icones anatomicae (1801)

Left: The frontispiece shows a cave with a pastoral dissection in progress. Despite the trappings of antiquity, Leopoldo Caldani was a modern man who conducted anatomical experiments with electricity. Above: Caldani, by an unknown artist.

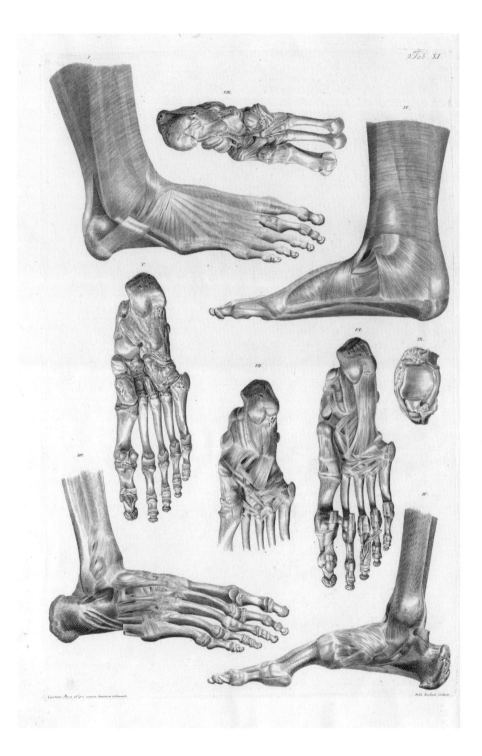

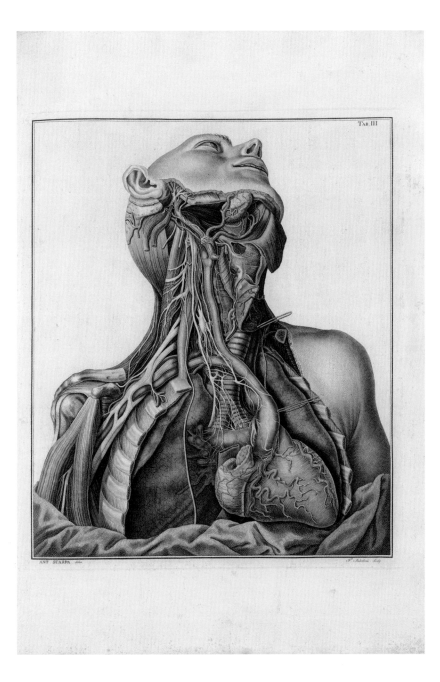

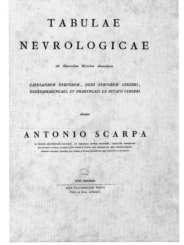

Tabulae neurologicae (1794)

Opposite: The complex muscles and skeleton of the foot. Left: The viscera and pulmonary system of the upper thorax and neck. Above: The title page. Overleaf: Hooks pull back the flesh to reveal the muscles and blood supply of the shoulder, neck and jaw.

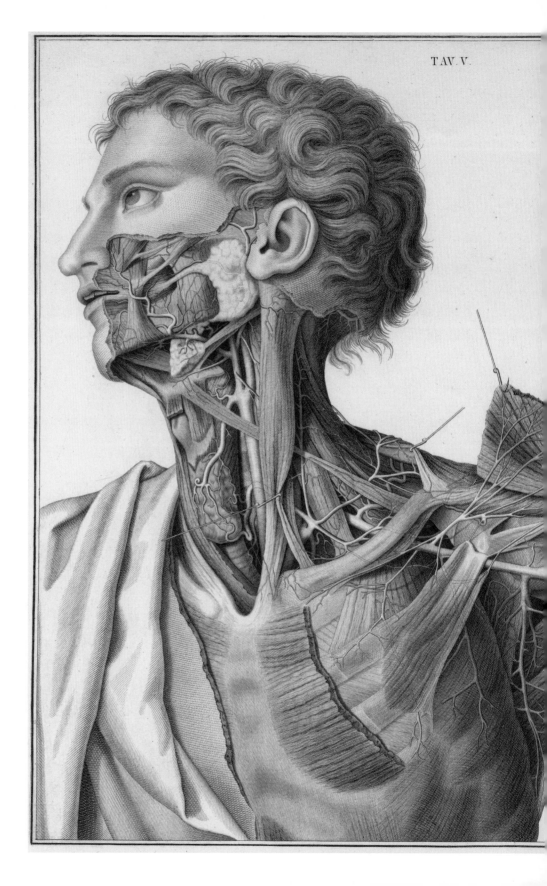

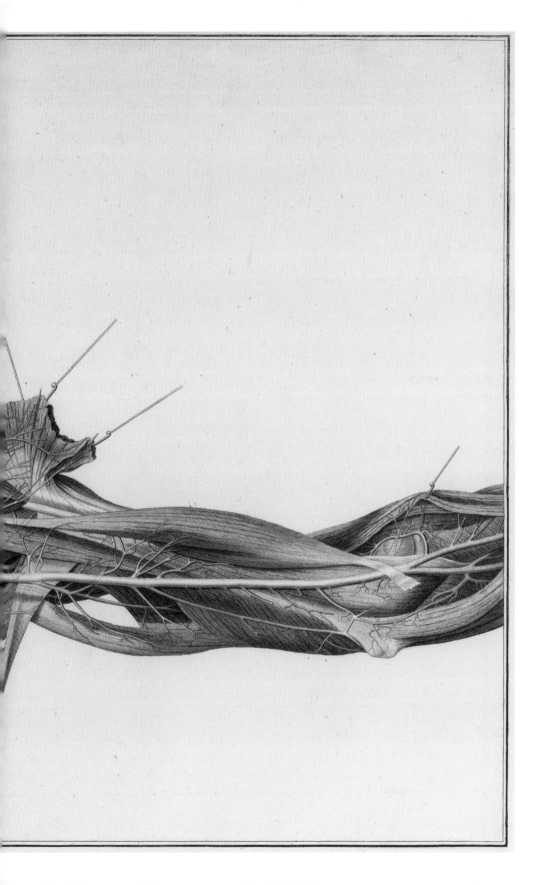

3 Xavier Bichat

In the same year that the first volume of Caldani's *Icones anatomicae* appeared (1801), Xavier Bichat's *Anatomie générale* (*General Anatomy*) was published. Bichat (1771–1802) achieved more in his short life than most do in a much longer one. The French Revolution erupted when he was just eighteen, and he served in its aftermath as a surgeon in the revolutionary Army of the Alps. The turmoil which enveloped France in the wake of that historic event hid Bichat's contributions to anatomy from the rest of the world for many years.

In his first book, published in 1800, he offered a completely new way of looking at the human anatomy. *Traité des membranes* (*Treatise on Membranes*) defined twenty-one different kinds of human tissue and argued that organs should be considered not as unique units but as different combinations of those tissues. He drew a comparison with chemistry, in which single elements combine to form compounds.

His next book, later the same year, *Recherches physiologiques sur la vie et la mort* (*Physiological Researches upon Life and Death*) addressed the consequences for pathology of such a view of the organs. In the intervening months Bichat had been appointed physician at the Hôtel-Dieu hospital in Paris, where he began to explore the impact of diseased tissue on the organs, and of medicines on the tissue. This was the first time that the effects of medicines had been studied scientifically. He dissected more than 600

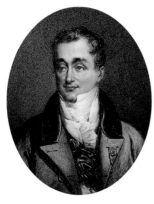

Xavier Bichat (1771–1802)

Above: Bichat planted the seeds of microscopic anatomy without the aid of a microscope. Right: The title page of Bichat's first book, *Traité des membranes* (1800); this edition is from 1816. Far right: The title page of *Anatomie générale* (1801).

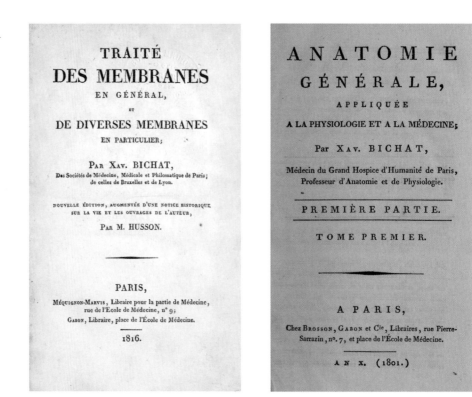

cadavers in six months, producing a large body of useful data which he discussed in both *Recherches physiologiques* and *Anatomie générale*. In his research Bichat developed the pathological ideas of Giovanni Morgagni and made a significant contribution to the science.

In *Recherches physiologiques* he attempted to define life in an anatomical sense; it was, he wrote, 'the totality of those set of functions which resist death'. Perhaps, with the benefit of his experience of the insanitary and bloody French Revolution, he continued, 'Such is the mode of existence of living bodies that everything surrounding them tends to destroy them.' It was no small irony that, surrounding himself with hundreds of diseased, decaying corpses, he eventually contracted typhoid and died only a year after *Anatomie générale* was published, at just thirty years old. He had been working on a new classification of diseases at the time.

Little known outside France at the time of his death, news of his work spread slowly to other countries; but the British author George Eliot in her 1872 novel *Middlemarch* writes admiringly of Bichat, and today his tissue doctrine marks the root of the science of histology – microscopic anatomy. Bichat's studies were all the more remarkable because he refused to use a microscope. What extraordinary discoveries he might have made had he lived longer and allowed himself to see his tissues at a cellular level.

The repercussions of the French Revolution were felt beyond the country's borders with the rest of Europe. When neighbouring states formed a coalition with the aim of supressing the revolt, France counter-attacked. In 1792 and again in 1797, French troops advanced into Germany as far as Mainz, where they remained in control until 1814.

4 Samuel Thomas von Sömmerring

Among those whom this displaced was the distinguished German anatomist Samuel Thomas von Sömmerring (1755–1830), dean of the university faculty of medicine in Mainz. He fled to Frankfurt, where he was an early advocate of vaccination against smallpox. He had already published several anatomical texts before he was invited to join the Bavarian Academy of Science in Munich in 1804. His description of cranial nerves, for example, is still used today, superseding successive earlier attempts by Galen, Vesalius, Fallopius, Eustachi and Thomas Willis; and with *Tabula sceleti feminine* (*A Chart of the Female Skeleton*), published in Frankfurt in 1795, he became the first man to describe accurately the different bone structure of a woman. He also wrote a paper on the anatomical danger of tightly laced bodices, which helped to bring an end to the late eighteenth-century fashion for impossibly thin waists.

Sömmerring marked the start of the nineteenth century with a series of four books on the sense organs: *Abbildungen des menschlichen Auges* (*Pictures of the Human Eye*, 1801), *Abbildungen des menschlichen Hörorgans* (*Pictures of the Human Ear*, 1806), *Abbildungen des menschlichen Organe des Geschmacks und der Stimme* (*Pictures of the Human Organ of Taste and Voice*, 1806) and *Abbildungen der menschlichen Organe des Geruchs* (*Pictures of the Human Organ of Smell*, 1809).

They were his final anatomical publications, and some of the most detailed studies of the organs yet produced. In Munich Sömmerring was distracted by other sciences. He wrote about fossil crocodiles and was the first to describe the pterodactyl. He designed an

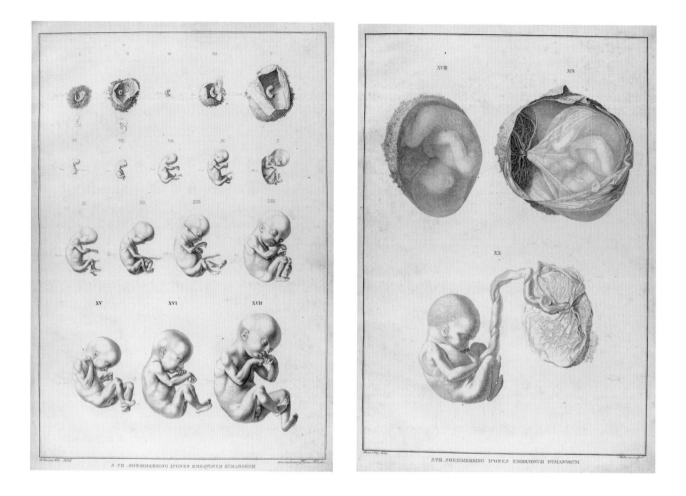

ABOVE

*Icones embryonum
humanorum* (1799)

Two pages from Thomas
Sömmerring's work, the first
to show the development of
the foetus.

astronomical telescope, and built Bavaria's first telegraph system, which is still preserved in the German Museum of Science in the city. At the age of sixty-five he began to find the Bavarian winters uncomfortable and retired to Frankfurt, his adoptive city, where he is remembered by his grave in the city cemetery and by Sömmerring's Wine Bar on Sömmerringstrasse.

5 Philipp Bozzini

Sömmerring the polymath played his part in both the advancement of anatomy and the flood of invention of the Science Age. The inventions of others directly transformed anatomy during the century, starting with Philipp Bozzini's ingenious device for seeing into human orifices without the need for a knife.

Bozzini (1773–1809) served as a surgeon in the Austrian army during the Coalition War against France. He was the physician for a large field hospital in Mainz, working around the clock in dark, difficult conditions to treat injured soldiers. A lack of light was sometimes the difference between life and death; so Bozzini designed an instrument which could not only introduce light into bodily cavities but allow them to be examined without having to perform exploratory surgery on an already injured patient. Light from a candle within the instrument was reflected down a steel tube with a variety of end attachments (specula) which could be inserted relatively painlessly into openings in the body. Bozzini had invented the first endoscope.

When the French army prevailed in Mainz, Bozzini (like Sömmerring) fled and made Frankfurt his home. Once his device had been licensed for medical use in 1806 he was a tireless promoter of it, which he called the *Lichtleiter* (light conductor). He introduced it to the world in a treatise in 1807: *Der Lichtleiter oder die Beschreibung einer einfachen Vorrichtung und ihrer Anwendung zur Erleuchtung innerer Höhlen und Zwischenräume des lebenden animalischen Körpers* (*The Light Conductor, or Description of a Simple Instrument and its Use for Illuminating Inner Cavities and Interstices of the Living Animal Body*), which deserves a place in the library.

Bozzini was a skilled draftsman and, like Sömmerring, he didn't confine his activities to anatomy. He was interested in chemistry; and, with echoes of Leonardo da Vinci, he is said to have used a good working knowledge of aeronautics to design a flying machine. He made his daily living in Frankfurt as a consultant obstetrician, during which his *Lichtleiter* will certainly have come into its own. He was one of Frankfurt's four official 'plague doctors', responsible for dealing with epidemics in the surrounding area; and, like Bichat, he died young of typhoid contracted in the execution of his duties.

Bozzini's *Lichtleiter* was far ahead of its time and would not be improved on for fifty years. Early attempts to harness electricity for light were made in the first half of the nineteenth century, but the first improvement to Bozzini's design was made by a French physician. In 1853 Antonin Jean Desormeaux replaced the candle with a brighter lamp which burned a mix of turpentine and alcohol. Desormeaux was the first to use an endoscope during minor surgical operations. A decade later Francis Cruise, a urologist in Dublin, made improvements to Desormeaux's device which he used during urethrotomies and other surgery.

Thomas Edison's invention of a reliable incandescent lightbulb in 1879 changed everyone's lives forever, by extending the working day into the hours of darkness. It transformed surgical practice and anatomical study, and the development of smaller bulbs made their use in endoscopy possible by the beginning of the twentieth century – a mere century after Bozzini.

6 Cadavers for dissection

By the beginning of the nineteenth century anatomy was firmly established as a vital part of training for surgery. In Britain this created two problems. Firstly, the number of anatomy schools naturally increased to cope with the demand from trainee surgeons; but there was no control over the quality of the teaching – students were merely required to attend two courses.

The Royal College of Surgeons began in 1822 to regulate schools with minimum standards and certification. The move was successful: uncertificated schools closed for lack of students and new schools with higher standards entered the market. A new law in

1858, the Medical Act, required all medical practitioners to be registered with the General Medical Council of the United Kingdom, which placed further stress on good medical education. By 1871 all but one of the country's anatomy schools were run by universities and attached to teaching hospitals.

The second problem, accompanying the rising number of anatomy students, was the falling number of cadavers legally available to be dissected. The Murder Act of 1752 had contributed to a reduction in the crime and therefore in the number of bodies executed for it and presented for dissection. The graverobbers who supplied anatomists in the eighteenth century continued to thrive in the early nineteenth. Although not all schools offered dissection as a teaching tool, in London alone some 475 bodies were being 'anatomised', most of them supplied by body snatchers. The source of such bodies was no secret, and there was even an agreed rate: a tutor could buy a child's body, for example, at six shillings (30p) for the first foot (30cm), and ninepence (3.3p) for each additional inch (2.54cm). Deformed or exceptional bodies attracted a considerably higher fee. It's no surprise that the public regarded the anatomy profession with distaste.

Sensational stories fuelled their antipathy. Graverobbing gangs formed in the major cities of the United Kingdom, each with their own patch. One such gang worked for eight reputable surgeons, stealing bodies from thirty churchyards, civic cemeteries and pauper burial grounds in the London borough of Lambeth. Such was the national

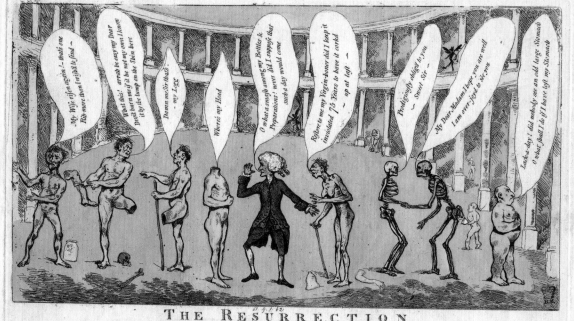

demand that gangs in London would export bodies to the rest of the country. On Liverpool docks in 1826, sailors investigating the smell coming from three large barrels discovered eleven bodies pickled in brine, labelled as 'bitter salts', on their way to Scotland's principal city, Edinburgh, whose anatomy school had a growing reputation at the time.

Some even resorted to murder to satisfy the demand for corpses. Edinburgh was the setting for the most famous case of body snatching, when William Burke and William Hare supplied anatomy tutor Robert Knox with at least sixteen bodies of men and women whom they had murdered for the purpose. They plied their victims with alcohol until they became helpless, then smothered them, a technique which became known as 'burking' and was taken up by other 'resurrectionists'. In London John Bishop and Thomas Williams were known as the London Burkers. Burking was undetectable on the anatomist's slab.

In Edinburgh Hare was acquitted for lack of evidence but Burke was hanged in 1829 in front of a crowd of 25,000 and his body sent for dissection. During it, Professor Monro from Edinburgh Medical School got out his pen and wrote on a scrap of paper, 'This is written with the blood of Wm Burke, who was hanged at Edinburgh. This blood was taken from his head.' The school preserved Burke's skeleton, which was exhibited in the city in a 2022 exhibition about the history of anatomy.

Many books have been written about Burke and Hare. The first, *The trial of William Burke and Helen M'Dougal: containing the whole legal proceedings against William Hare, in order to bring him to trial for the murder of James Wilson, or Daft Jamie. With an appendix of curious and interesting information, regarding the late West-Port murders*, appeared within weeks of the trial, from shorthand records taken at the hearing by one John Macnee. It sold so well that a *Supplement to the Trial* was published soon afterwards, containing anything else about the murders that the writer and publisher could justify.

The case has inspired speculative crime authors ever since. The noted Scottish playwright James Bridie's play *The Anatomist*, a comedy based on Burke and Hare's exploits, received its premiere in 1931. However, only one book can claim a very direct connection with William Burke. In the possession of the Royal College of Surgeons in Edinburgh is a small notebook, bound in the skin of the man himself. The cover has been printed in gold with the words 'Burke's Skin Pocket Book' and a decorative border, and on the back someone has noted, 'Executed 28 Jan 1829.'

Despite the public outrage at the Edinburgh murders, the practice of bodysnatching continued unabated. Further north in Scotland, in 1831, a dog unearthed a body which had been carelessly buried after its dissection in the anatomy theatre of Aberdeen's King's College. As word spread, a crowd of 100 or so gathered to protest. Some broke into the college, where they found three further bodies prepared for study, and the unfortunate Dr Andrew Moir, the city's first anatomy lecturer, whom they assaulted and chased down the street. The crowd, by now swollen to around 20,000, then burned the building to the ground with shouts of, 'Down with the burking shop!'

Demonstrations such as these persuaded the British government to act, and in 1832 it passed the Anatomy Act, which broadened the source of bodies which could be dissected. It ended the use of executed criminals, which had been enabled by the Murder Act of

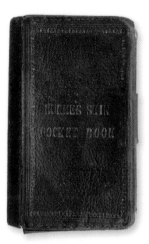

ABOVE

Burke's Skin Pocket Book (1829)

A small souvenir notebook bound in the skin of the Edinburgh grave robber William Burke.

1752, but made it legal to procure the remains of the deceased poor from Britain's charitable hospitals and workhouses, provided they had not been claimed by friends or relatives within forty-eight hours of death.

The Act was successful, particularly after the passing of the Poor Law Amendment Act of 1834 which drove more paupers into the workhouses. Conditions in these overcrowded, underfunded institutions declined, resulting in even more deaths and more bodies for dissection. Workhouse directors sold bodies to recoup expenses, and this legal trade drove down the price of now readily available cadavers to the point where it was eventually no longer viable for the resurrectionists to deal illegally. The effect was akin to the legalisation of banned drugs.

The Anatomy Act also had the effect of highlighting Britain's notorious class system. The rich, the powerful and the highly educated all supported dissection because it advanced science; but it was never their bodies being dissected. The corpses left unclaimed at the workhouse were those of people who had entered it impoverished and whose families could not afford to bury them. The unintended consequence of the Anatomy Act was to make the humiliating, desecrating public dissection of one's corpse an unwelcome preserve of the poor. Dissection was no longer a punishment for crime, but a punishment for being poor.

7 Jones, Richard and Sir Richard Quain

The Royal College of Surgeons' move to regulate anatomy education prompted a demand for modern students' textbooks. Two Irish brothers and their cousin all published useful teaching books for the profession.

Jones Quain (1796–1865), the elder of the brothers, moved from County Cork to London in 1825 and got a post at Aldersgate Medical School, which had opened that year as a deliberate act of defiance of the Royal College of Surgeons' (RCS) new policy. It proved to be one of the better private schools, which became its undoing – gradually its teaching staff were headhunted by rival institutions, and the school itself closed in 1848. Despite his protest, the school's founder, William Lawrence, eventually became president of the RCS. Quain, who himself joined the RCS in 1825, was appointed Professor of General Anatomy at University College, London (UCL), in 1831.

His teaching experiences at Aldersgate prompted Jones Quain to write *Elements of Descriptive and Practical Anatomy for the Use of Students*, which was published in 1828 and quickly established itself as a standard teaching text. It was regularly updated throughout the century and ran to ten editions over the following sixty years, the last four revised posthumously. It was not rivalled until Henry Gray's *Anatomy* arrived in 1858.

Jones' younger brother Richard Quain (1800–87) was briefly a student of Jones at Aldersgate, then took up a post as anatomy demonstrator at UCL in 1828. He was, again briefly, his brother's demonstrator there; but a year later, in 1832, Richard was offered the

The Anatomy of the Arteries (1844)

Below: The title page of the book by Richard Quain (1800–87). Opposite: A dissection of the abdomen, with the right hand pulled out of the way by a bandage. The sketchy representation of the surrounding shroud emphasises the precision of the anatomical detail. Overleaf left: A head leant backward over a wooden block exposes the anatomy of the neck and lower jaw. Overleaf right: The anatomy of the cheek.

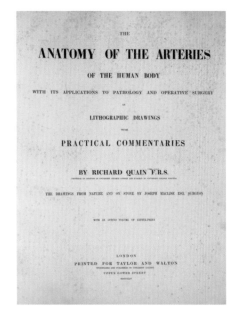

THE

ANATOMY OF THE ARTERIES

OF THE HUMAN BODY

WITH ITS APPLICATIONS TO PATHOLOGY AND OPERATIVE SURGERY

IN

LITHOGRAPHIC DRAWINGS

WITH

PRACTICAL COMMENTARIES

BY RICHARD QUAIN F.R.S.

THE DRAWINGS FROM NATURE AND ON STONE BY JOSEPH MACLISE ESQ. SURGEON

LONDON
PRINTED FOR TAYLOR AND WALTON

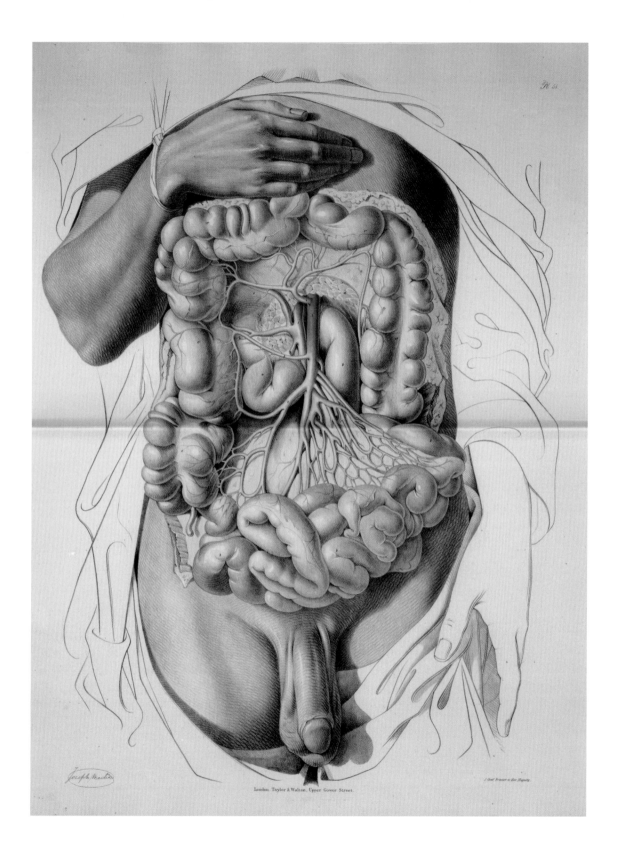

Pl. 34.

Joseph Maclise

London, Taylor & Walton, Upper Gower Street.

J. Graf, Printer to Her Majesty.

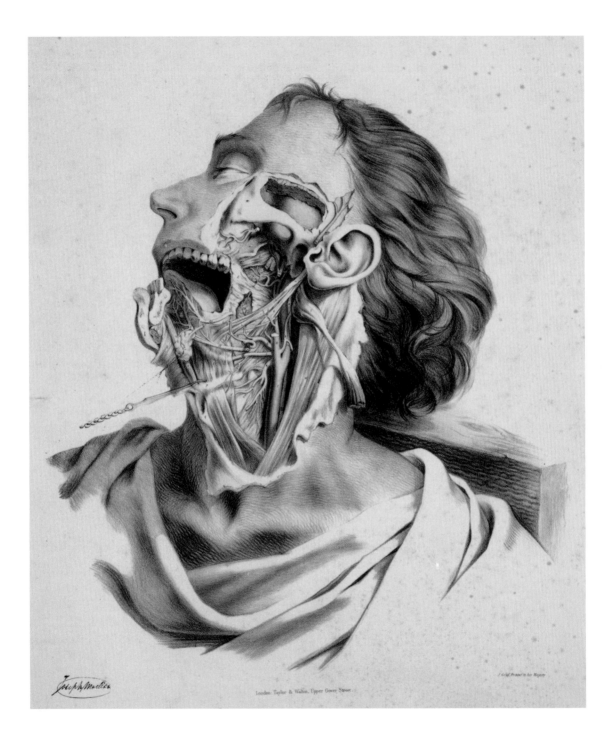

Joseph Maclise

London. Taylor & Walton, Upper Gower Street.

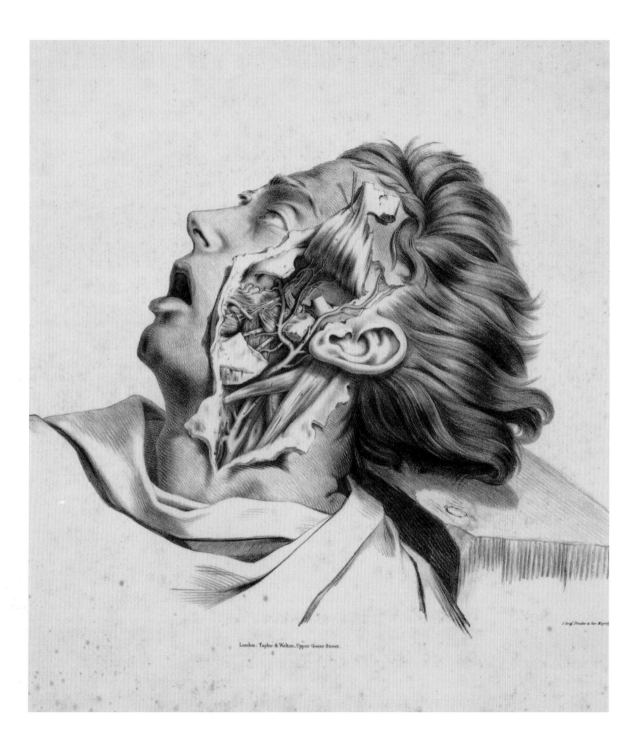

London: Taylor & Walton, Upper Gower Street.

J. Graf, Printer to her Majesty

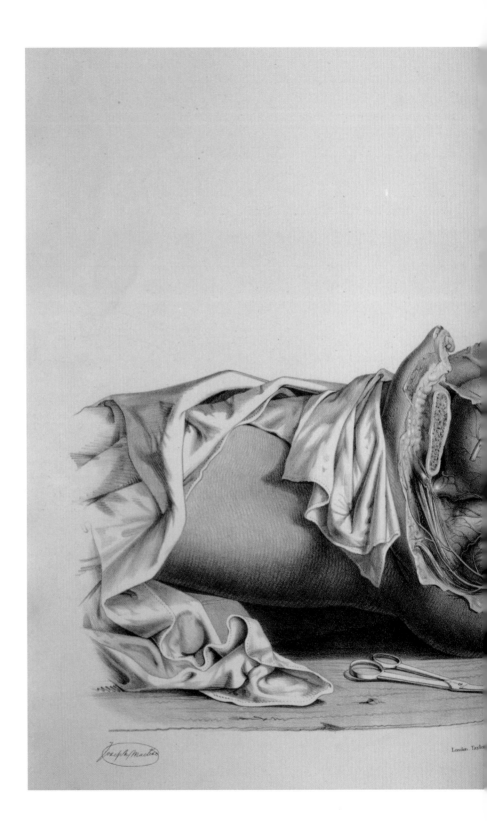

Joseph Maclise

London: Taylor

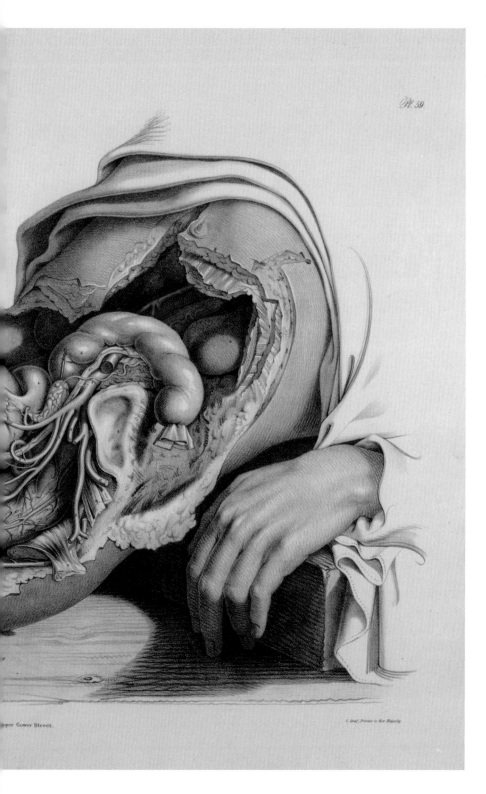

Pl. 50.

per Gower Street.

C. Graf, Printer to Her Majesty.

LEFT

Anatomy of the Arteries (1844)

Joseph Maclise's drawings
for Richard Quain's book
are exquisite in artistry, here
including cross-sections of
tissue in a view of the viscera of
a female pelvis.

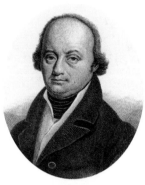

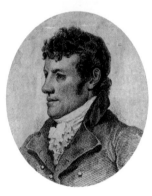

chair in Descriptive Anatomy at UCL, and eventually rose to become Special Professor of Clinical Surgery at the university's North London Teaching Hospital. His progress was sometimes hampered by his bad temper and his jealousy of the success of others, whom he often accused of having ulterior motives. If he resented his older brother's advancement, it did not prevent him from editing the 1848 edition of Jones's *Elements of Descriptive and Practical Anatomy.*

Richard Quain published his own highly acclaimed book, *The Anatomy of the Arteries of the Human Body, with its Applications to Pathology and Operative Surgery* in 1844. It was based on his observations of some 1,040 dissections. The drawings were by another Irishman working in London, the artist Joseph Maclise. While still realistic representations of a dissected corpse, they tend to the diagrammatical by softening the lines of the less relevant areas of the body surrounding the area of interest, a technique which focusses the viewer's eye on the parts that matter. It is a beautiful book.

The annotations for Maclise's plates were written by another Richard Quain, Jones' and Richard's cousin. This Richard Quain eventually served Queen Victoria as physician-extraordinary and the ensuing baronetcy entitled him to be addressed as Sir Richard.

Sir Richard Quain (1816–98) was almost certainly taught anatomy by his cousin Richard at UCL, where he enrolled to study medicine in 1837. In time, he was appointed to the role his cousin Jones had once occupied, as Professor of General Anatomy at UCL. He resigned in 1850, however, to concentrate on his lucrative physician's practice, which included posts as consulting physician at three hospitals in the south of England.

Sir Richard broke new ground in medical publishing with *Quain's Dictionary of Medicine,* of which he was editor and a contributor. Seven years in the compilation, it was – in 1882 – the first such volume, filling a significant gap in the medical student's armoury and remaining in print into the twentieth century. He is remembered in physiology for an article on fatty diseases of the heart which he wrote in 1850, and which has led to one condition being known as Quain's fatty heart.

8 Phrenology

The progress of anatomy has been one of dispelling myths and discovering the truth about the structures of the human body. Very rarely, at least in the modern era, has it gone down a blind alley. Yet a curious fad gripped the medical community in the first half of the nineteenth century – phrenology. The idea that one could detect an individual's personality by the bumps on their skull was based on flawed anatomical reasoning and was debunked by the middle of the century; but its rapid popularisation and a lingering belief in it, even today, should serve as a reminder of the importance of scientific rigour.

German physician Franz Joseph Gall (1758–1828) had been fascinated even in childhood about the differences in character between the various members of his family. In 1796 he began to lecture on the subject, based on his own theories. He believed that the brain consisted of several different 'muscles', each responsible for a different aspect of behaviour, and that each 'muscle' could be over- or under-developed, giving rise to irregularities of the surface of the skull. He published his ideas in *Anatomie et physiologie du système nerveux en général, et du cerveau en particulier, avec des observations sur la possibilité reconnoitre plusieurs dispositions intellectuelles et morales de l'homme et des animaux, par la configuration de leurs têtes* (*The Anatomy and Physiology of the Nervous System in General, and of the Brain in Particular, with Observations upon the possibility of ascertaining the several Intellectual and Moral Dispositions of Man and Animal, by the configuration of their Heads*), in 1819.

Gall and his assistant Johann Gaspar Spurzheim (1776–1832) had earlier co-written *Untersuchungen über die Anatomie des Nervensystems überhaupt, und des Gehirns insbesondere* (*Investigations into the Anatomy of the Nervous System in General, and of the Brain in Particular*), published in 1809. But the two men disagreed about the nature and implications of this new 'science' and Spurzheim began his own lecture series, 'The Physiognomical System of Drs Gall and Spurzheim'. It was Spurzheim who coined the word phrenology; and where Gall recognised twenty-seven different 'muscles', Spurzheim identified forty. He travelled widely throughout Europe, popularising the idea of phrenology. The often-reproduced, white ceramic heads with the different phrenological regions of the brain mapped on them are based on visual aids that Spurzheim used to make his points.

Edinburgh in Scotland became a particular centre of study after Spurzheim visited the city in person in 1816 to refute a journal article critical of the theory. France took enthusiastically to phrenology and several French works on the subject were published, most notably *Traité de phrénologie humaine et comparée* (*Treatise of Human and Comparative Phrenology*) by Joseph Vimont (1795–1857). This was a large volume

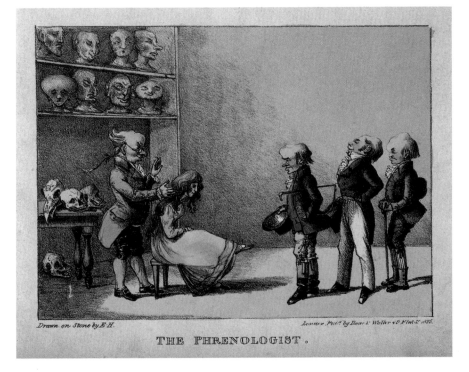

THE PHRENOLOGIST.

LEFT

The Phrenologist (1825)

Edward Hull (active 1820–34) lampoons the craze for phrenology in an image of a group of phrenologists with oddly shaped skulls examining the head of a young woman.

Franz Joseph Gall
(1758–1828)

An illustration from a French
edition of Gall's theory of
phrenology. Below his portrait,
three skulls indicate the
supposed correlation between
irregular bumps on the head
and character traits.

Traité de phrénologie humaine
et comparée (1832)

The skull of a child with
hydrocephalus, a build-up of
fluid in the brain, from Joseph
Vimont's book on phrenology.

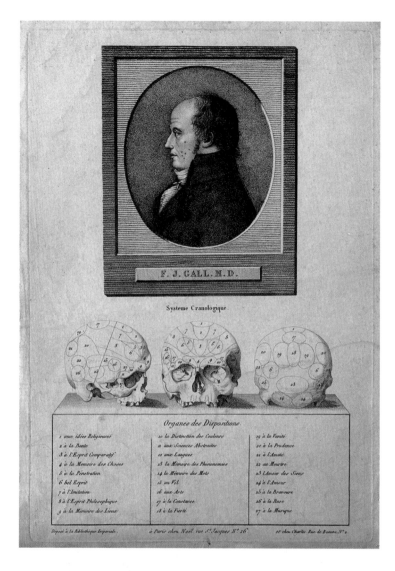

containing life-size images of human and animal skulls by noted lithographer Godefroy
Engelmann. Aware of its market potential, its publisher issued the first volume, in 1832,
with parallel French and English text and captions.

Phrenology was also popular in the United States, and Spurzheim undertook a lecture
tour there in 1832. The tour was cut short by his death in Boston of typhoid; such was
his popularity that Bostonians removed his brain, skull and heart for preservation and
display, held an elaborate funeral and erected a monumental sarcophagus to his memory
in a Massachusetts cemetery.

There is no correlation between bumps on the head and character. Spurzheim argued

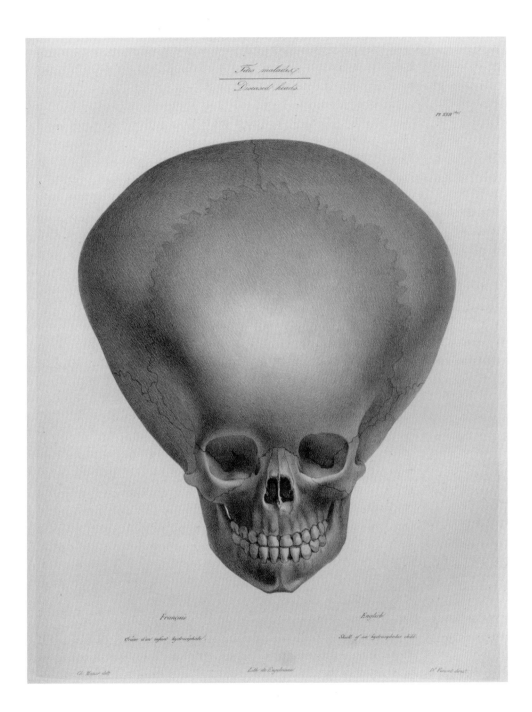

Diseased heads.

Pl XXII

Français

Crâne d'un enfant hydrocéphale.

English

Skull of an hydrocephalic child.

Ch. Mercier delt.

Lith. de Engelmann

Dr Vincent sculpt.

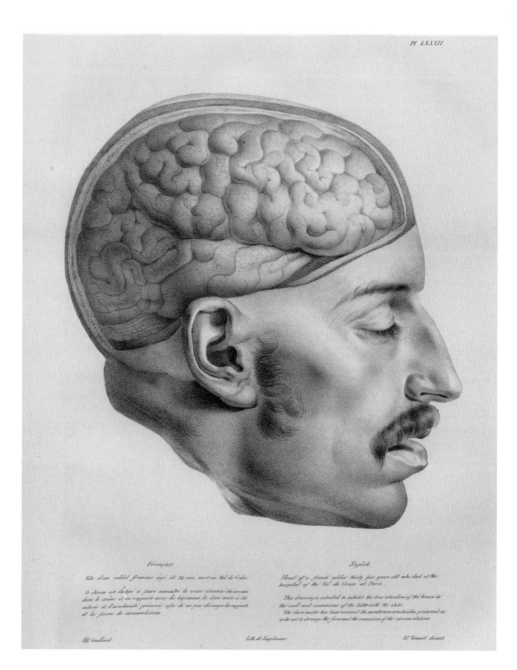

that there was, and that there was a hierarchy about the bumps. The inference was that the shape of one's skull somehow embodied an innate superiority or inferiority, something which endeared phrenology and other pseudo-sciences to those with racist, sexist or intellectualist agendas and has ensured renewed interest in it from time to time ever since.

Although Franz Joseph Gall's science was weak, he does deserve credit for being one of the first to suggest that different areas of the brain had different roles. It was a Frenchman working in the same field, Pierre Paul Broca (1824–80), who did much to disprove the theory of phrenology. His work on the region of the brain associated with speech, known today as Broca's area, was the first rigorously scientific proof of localisation of brain function. Broca exhibited his own scientific racism in believing at first that Black people were an intermediate stage between apes and humans, something he came to reject in later life.

Broca first published his studies on speech and the brain as *Remarques sur le siège de la faculté du langage articulé* (*Remarks on the Seat of the Function of Spoken Language*) in the *Bulletin de la Société Anatomique de Paris* in 1861. The breakthrough had additional resonance coming just two years after Charles Darwin's book *On the Origin of Species*. Although Darwin (1809–82) wasn't an anatomist, his theory of evolution had implications for all branches of the life sciences.

OPPOSITE

Traité de phrénologie humaine et compare (1832)

The head of a French soldier, showing 'the true situation of the brain in the scull and the connexions of the latter with the skin'.

9 Henry Gray

Of more immediate interest to anatomists, in the year before Darwin's entrance into public life, was the publication of the one anatomy book that everyone knows. *Anatomy: Descriptive and Surgical*, or by its more familiar title *Gray's Anatomy*, is now in its forty-second edition, all forty-two of them occupying several shelves in the anatomist's library. It is surely the longest-running anatomy title in a practical rather than merely historical context. All but the first two editions were published after Gray's early death from smallpox, a measure of the abiding usefulness of his book.

Gray (1827–61) showed promise as a medical student at St George's teaching hospital in London. He was a product of the RCS's drive to raise standards of education and of the 1832 Anatomy Act which improved the supply of cadavers for dissection. Gray was known as a careful anatomist and an acute observer and won a prize in 1848 awarded by the RCS for a treatise on the comparative anatomy of vertebrate eyes.

He was employed as a lecturer at St George's in 1853, where he saw a need for a low-priced, well-organised anatomy textbook for his students. To that end he worked with Henry Vandyke Carter, a former dissector at St George's with whom Gray had already collaborated on a paper about spleen. Carter drew the illustrations for *Gray's Anatomy* and deserves much of the credit for its success. The publisher of the first edition originally intended this by printing both men's names in the same size of font; but, at Gray's insistence, Carter's was reduced and his credential as Professor of Anatomy of Grant College in Bombay deleted, leaving only a description as 'late demonstrator of anatomy.'

Gray had previously failed to acknowledge Carter at all in their paper on spleen, for which Gray had won a prize of 300 guineas. Gray received a three-shilling royalty for

terminates on the left side, in the thoracic duct; on the right side, in the right lymphatic duct.

229.—The Deep Lymphatics and Glands of the Neck and Thorax.

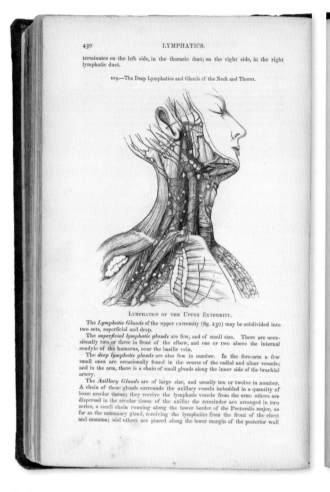

LYMPHATICS OF THE UPPER EXTREMITY.

The *Lymphatic Glands* of the upper extremity (fig. 230) may be subdivided into two sets, superficial and deep.

The *superficial lymphatic glands* are few, and of small size. There are occasionally two or three in front of the elbow, and one or two above the internal condyle of the humerus, near the basilic vein.

The *deep lymphatic glands* are also few in number. In the fore-arm a few small ones are occasionally found in the course of the radial and ulnar vessels; and in the arm, there is a chain of small glands along the inner side of the brachial artery.

The *Axillary Glands* are of large size, and usually ten or twelve in number. A chain of these glands surrounds the axillary vessels imbedded in a quantity of loose areolar tissue; they receive the lymphatic vessels from the arm; others are dispersed in the areolar tissue of the axilla: the remainder are arranged in two series, a small chain running along the lower border of the Pectoralis major, as far as the mammary gland, receiving the lymphatics from the front of the chest and mamma; and others are placed along the lower margin of the posterior wall

in the deep cervical glands. They have not at present been demonstrated in the dura mater, or in the substance of the brain.

The *Lymphatic Glands of the Neck* are divided into two sets, superficial and deep.

The *superficial cervical glands* are placed in the course of the external jugular vein, between the Platysma and Sterno-mastoid. They are most numerous at the root of the neck, in the triangular interval between the clavicle, the Sterno-mastoid, and the Trapezius, where they are continuous with the axillary glands. A few small glands are also found on the front and sides of the larynx.

228.—The Superficial Lymphatics and Glands of the Head, Face, and Neck.

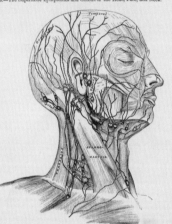

The *deep cervical glands* (fig. 229) are numerous and of large size; they form an uninterrupted chain along the sheath of the carotid artery and internal jugular vein, lying by the side of the pharynx, œsophagus, and trachea, and extending from the base of the skull to the thorax, where they communicate with the lymphatic glands in this cavity.

The *Superficial and Deep Cervical Lymphatics* are a continuation of those already described on the cranium and face. After traversing the glands in those regions, they pass through the chain of glands which lie along the sheath of the carotid vessels, being joined by the lymphatics from the pharynx, œsophagus, larynx, trachea, and thyroid gland. At the lower part of the neck, after receiving some lymphatics from the thorax, they unite into a single trunk, which

Gray's Anatomy (1858)

Simple clear line drawings by Henry Vandyke Carter were key to the early success of Henry Gray's *Anatomy Descriptive and Surgical*. From left to right: The deep lymphatics and glands of the neck and thorax. The superficial lymphatics and glands of the head, face and neck. The nerves of the scalp, face and side of the neck. The superficial lymphatics and glands of the upper extremity.

The *Temporo-facial*, the larger of the two terminal branches, passes upwards and forwards through the parotid gland, crosses the neck of the condyle of the jaw, being connected in this situation with the auriculo-temporal branch of the inferior maxillary nerve, and divides into branches, which are distributed over the temple and upper part of the face; these may be divided into three sets, temporal, malar, and infra-orbital.

The *temporal branches* cross the zygoma to the temporal region, supplying the Attrahens aurem and the integument, and join with the temporal branch of the superior maxillary, and with the auriculo-temporal branch of the inferior maxillary. The more anterior branches supply the frontal portion of the Occipito-

255.—The Nerves of the Scalp, Face, and Side of the Neck.

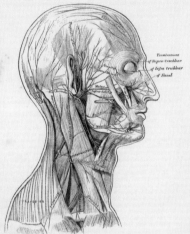

frontalis, and the Orbicularis palpebrarum muscle, joining with the supra-orbital branch of the ophthalmic.

The *malar branches* pass across the malar bone to the outer angle of the orbit, where they supply the Orbicularis and Corrugator supercilii muscles, joining with filaments from the lachrymal and supra-orbital nerves: others supply the lower eyelid, joining with filaments of the malar branches of the superior maxillary nerve.

The *infra-orbital*, of larger size than the rest, pass horizontally forwards to

of the axilla, which receive the lymphatics from the integument of the back. Two or three subclavian lymphatic glands are placed immediately beneath the clavicle; it is through these that the axillary and deep cervical glands communicate with each other. One is figured by Mascagni near the umbilicus. In malignant diseases, tumours or other affections implicating the upper part of the back and shoulder, the front of the chest and mamma, the upper part of the front and side of the abdomen, or the hand, fore-arm, and arm, these glands are usually found enlarged.

232.—The Superficial Lymphatics and Glands of the Upper Extremity.

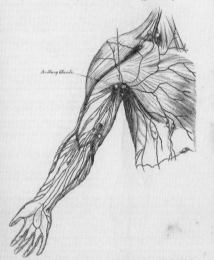

The *Superficial Lymphatics* of the upper extremity arise from the skin of the hand, and run along the sides of the fingers chiefly on the dorsal surface of the hand; they then pass up the fore-arm, and subdivide into two sets, which take the course of the subcutaneous veins. Those from the inner border of the hand accompany the ulnar veins along the inner side of the fore-arm to the bend of the elbow, where they join with some lymphatics from the outer side of the fore-arm, follow the course of the basilic vein, communicate with the glands imme-

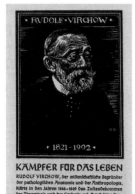

ABOVE

Rudolf Virchow (1821–1902)

A woodcut portrait of Virchow, 'Fighter for Life', the father of cellular pathology.

each copy of *Gray's Anatomy* sold, while Carter was paid only a one-off fee of £150. Although the two men are usually portrayed as friends, there are references to Gray in Carter's diaries as a 'snob', and as motivated by 'jealousy, p'raps'. Carter's clear illustrations were used in successive editions of the book for the next sixty years.

There were 363 of them in the first edition, which was 750 pages in length. The book was popular because of the clarity of its drawings and the breadth of its coverage. It was a useful reference book for professionals as well as a guide for beginners. In an effort to maintain its reputation as an all-encompassing authority, later editors of *Gray's Anatomy* added more and more sections to it, to the extent that the comprehensive thirty-eighth edition (1990) ran to 2,092 pages.

Since then, some effort has been made to return to its educational roots; but the fact that it has spawned companion volumes such as *Gray's Anatomy for Students* and *Gray's Atlas of Anatomy* shows how embedded in the medical profession the book has become. Carter's illustrations may have given way to successive technologies such as photography and online three-dimensional models; and Gray's systemic approach was replaced – although only as recently as the thirty-ninth edition – by a regional one. But its reputation and position seem unassailable.

10 Rudolf Virchow

Arriving in 1858, *Gray's Anatomy* was timely. The same year saw the enactment of the Medical Act, 'an Act to regulate the Qualifications of Practitioners in Medicine and Surgery ... Whereas it is expedient that Persons requiring Medical Aid should be enabled to distinguish qualified from unqualified Practitioners.' The year also saw the publication of Rudolf Virchow's *Die Cellularpathologie in ihrer Begründung auf physiologische und pathologische Gewebelehre* (*Cellular Pathology as Based upon Physiological and Pathological Histology*), a significant advance in anatomy which would only be reflected in later editions of Henry Gray's book.

Virchow (1821–1902) is the pathologist that Xavier Bichat could have been if only he had embraced the use of the microscope. Where Bichat was only able to see and understand the tissue of which organs are composed, Virchow saw into the cells of which tissue is formed. He studied the ways in which they changed with disease, and *Cellularpathologie* is no less than the beginning of a new phase of applied anatomy – histology.

From now on the important breakthroughs in anatomy would be made at this cellular level. As Virchow wrote in his book, 'all cells come from cells,' an echo of the Italian biologist Francesco Redi who declared that 'every living thing comes from a living thing.' It was a counter to the popular belief that lower forms of life simply emerged spontaneously from their environment – for example, that maggots were a product of rotting flesh rather than hatching from eggs laid by flies, as we now know.

Rudolf Virchow's first publication was a paper in 1845 containing the earliest pathological description of leukaemia, a condition which he also named (from the Greek for 'white blood'). He became convinced that diseases were the result of changes in previously healthy cells, and that different sets of cells were affected by different types of disease. At a time when doctors formed diagnoses based entirely on symptoms, Virchow argued that they might reach more accurate conclusions by examining diseased cells. He devoted his life to studying disease, describing and naming many of them for the first time – thrombosis, embolism, chordoma, ochronosis and more.

Not all doctors like to be told that what they are doing is wrong; and Virchow met with considerable opposition to his ideas. Journals refused to publish his papers, an obstacle which he overcame by launching his own. *Archiv für pathologische Anatomie und Physiologie, und für klinische Medizin* (*The Archive for Pathological Anatomy and Physiology and Clinical Medicine*), determinedly modern in approach and insistent on rigorous research, is still published today as a monthly peer-reviewed journal now called *Virchows Archiv: European Journal of Pathology*.

He was that most powerful advocate for public health, a physician and a politician. He was shocked by the poverty he witnessed when he visited a region of his native Germany struck by an outbreak of typhoid. 'Medicine is a social science,' he declared,

BELOW
Die Cellularpathologie (1858)

Left: Calcified cartilage in the tibia of seven-month foetus, at two levels of magnification. Right: The ovary of a frog, containing ova at various stages of development.

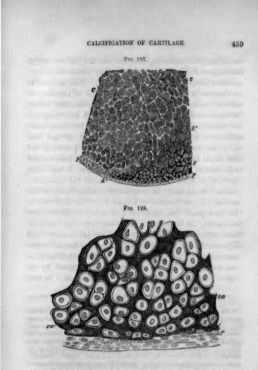

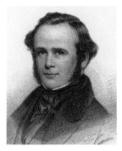

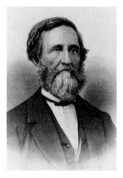

TOP
Horace Wells (1815–48)

Wells demonstrated anaesthesia using nitrous oxide in 1845.

ABOVE
Crawford Long (1815–78)

Long demonstrated anaesthesia using diethyl ether in 1846.

RIGHT
The First Use of Ether in Dental Surgery (1846)

A painting by Ernest Board (1877–1934) shows William Morton anaesthetising a patient in front of an invited audience. The painting is part of a series depicting medical milestones which Board painted for the philanthropist Henry Wellcome.

'and politics is nothing else but medicine on a large scale.' Virchow was sacked for taking part in the wave of attempted socialist revolutions which swept through Europe in 1848, and later co-founded the Deutsche Fortschrittspartei (German Progress Party). His opposition to Otto von Bismarck's military budget resulted in the latter challenging him to a duel. There are two versions of the outcome of the challenge. The most likely is that Virchow declined on the grounds that duelling was uncivilised. Another, however, claims that, as the person challenged, Virchow had the choice of weapons. He chose two sausages – one safe to eat, the other containing parasitic roundworm larvae. In this version, it was Bismarck who declined.

Virchow's first career choice was to become a Protestant pastor, a calling in which he graduated with a thesis entitled *Ein Leben voller Arbeit und Mühe ist keine Last, sondern eine Wohlthat* (*A Life Full of Work and Toil is not a Burden but a Benediction*). It may be said that he lived his life by that maxim. He died not of any disease but of a general decline in his health after breaking a leg jumping from a moving tram at the age of eighty-one.

11 Anaesthetics

Anatomy continued to benefit from invention in the second half of the century. After Hanaoka Seishū's mastectomy with his *tsūsensan* in 1804, it was more than forty years before anyone in the west successfully operated on an anaesthetised patient. A Massachusetts dentist Horace Wells (1815–48) gave a public demonstration in Boston of anaesthesia using nitrous oxide in 1845; but he underestimated the dose required and his patient complained loudly of the pain.

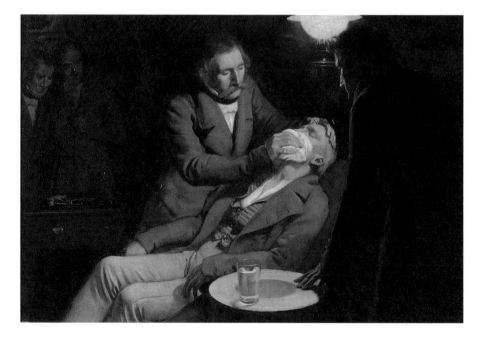

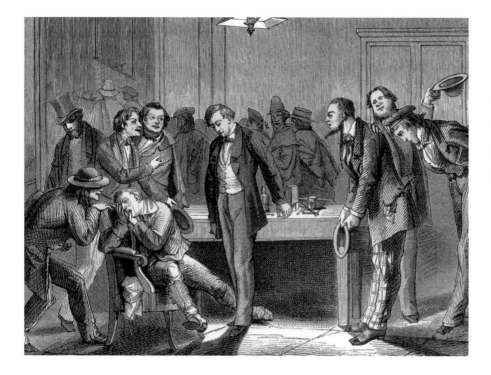

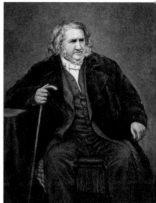

In 1846 an American surgeon in Georgia, Crawford Long (1815–78), removed two tumours from a student who had been anaesthetised with diethyl ether. Long had seen the student, with others, indulging in what they called 'ether frolics' – inhaling diethyl ether, under the influence of which they stumbled about, often injuring themselves but feeling no pain.

Later the same year, Horace Wells's partner in dental practice William Morton (1819–68), unaware of Long's success, demonstrated diethyl ether in Boston's Massachusetts General Hospital by administering it to a patient and then removing a tumour from their neck. The surgeon involved, sceptical before the operation, turned to observers afterwards and told them, 'Gentlemen, this is no humbug.' The theatre in which the operation took place is today called the Ether Dome. A Scottish obstetrician James Young Simpson (1811–70) first demonstrated the efficacy of chloroform on a human patient in 1847, and the substance soon replaced ether, which was highly flammable and often induced vomiting.

The safe use of anaesthetics made surgery an elective option, not just an emergency one. Surgical procedures could now be conducted in a measured way, not in a life-saving rush. Of greatest benefit to the pure science of anatomy, if not necessarily to the patient, was the new possibility of observing the internal systems and organs of a living body. This had previously only been possible, and impractically so, in the thick of battle or in the aftermath of gladiatorial combat.

12 Refrigeration

One of the oldest problems facing anatomy students and their teachers was the putrefaction of their cadavers, which made classes in dissection only tolerable in the cold winter months. One of the inventions most beneficial to anatomy was, therefore, refrigeration. Individual organs and other samples could be preserved in jars of spirit, but to treat a whole cadaver in the same way was impractical. Ferdinand Carré in France and Carl von Linde in Germany both worked on refrigeration in the 1860s, but the first use of freezing in anatomy used a much older method.

Christian Wilhelm Braune was a professor of anatomy at the University of Leipzig who froze bodies by sealing them in a waterproof box, placing the box in a larger tank and surrounding it with a mixture of ice and salt. Over a period of five days this could reduce the temperature inside the box to as little as $-21°C$ ($-5.8°F$); a human corpse freezes solid at $-18°C$ ($-0.4°F$). Braune (1831–92) then used a fine-toothed saw to slice sections of the body. Since the action of the saw raised the temperature, it took great skill to do so without tearing any tissue.

Braune's slices were thick by today's standards. Horizontal sections, from left to right across the body, were 2–3cm (¾–1¼in) deep; vertical ones from front to back thicker still. They could be studied still frozen (when it was possible to trace the details directly and accurately onto paper or glass laid over the section); or thawed, then either hardened with alcohol or preserved in spirit for display. The technique offered a new perspective on anatomical detail, anticipating the CT scan images to which we are accustomed today. Braune's book *Topographisch-anatomischer Atlas: nach Durchschnitten an gefrorenen Cadavern* (*Topographical Anatomy Atlas: from Cross-Sections of Frozen Cadavers*) was a sensation when it was published in 1867. It became the most popular anatomy textbook in Germany, and inspired others to experiment with the process.

Braune followed his Atlas with *Die Lage des Uterus und Fötus am Ende der Schwangerschaft nach Durchschnitten an gefrorenen Kadavern* (*The Position of the Uterus and Foetus at the End of Pregnancy from Cross-Sections of Frozen Cadavers*) in 1873. The images in this were based on an unfortunate young woman who had hanged herself in the final stages of her term, and whose body Braune had received and frozen in 1870. Braune bisected mother and child from top to bottom, but then reunited the two halves of the foetus.

13 Embalming

One long-standing solution to preservation was to embalm a corpse. The practice is at least 8,000 years old, as the artificially mummified remains of the Chinchorro people of the Atacama Desert testify. Alexander the Great was embalmed in honey in order to return his body from Babylon to Alexandria. Embalming was at its ceremonial height in Ancient Egypt, but as anatomy became more popular in Europe (and suitable cadavers relatively harder to come by) embalming was a very practical requirement. Many early anatomists injected wax into bodies; and, for a period, arsenic was considered a key ingredient of embalming fluid.

The eighteenth-century brothers William and John Hunter were the first of the modern age to develop oils which could be injected into the blood vessels and cavities of

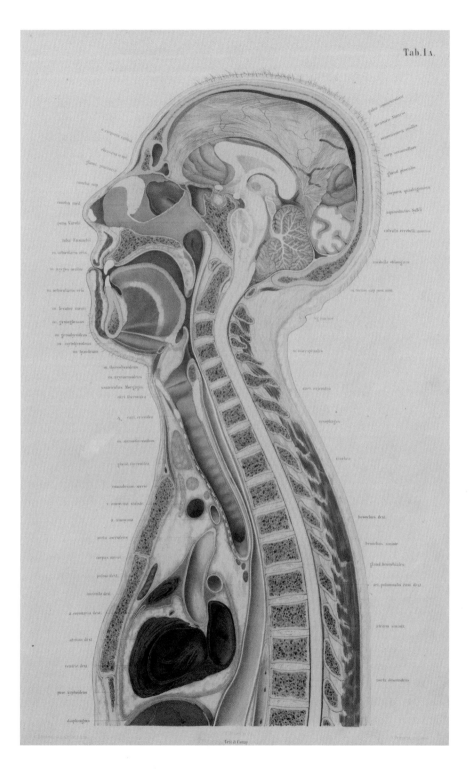

Tab. Iᴀ.

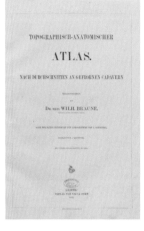

***Topographisch-anatomischer
Atlas*** (1867)

Left: A section of the head
and thorax sawn from a
frozen cadaver, in a plate by
C. Schmiedel from Christian
Wilhelm Braune's *Atlas*. Above:
The title page of the book,
which presented anatomy in a
new two-dimensional format.

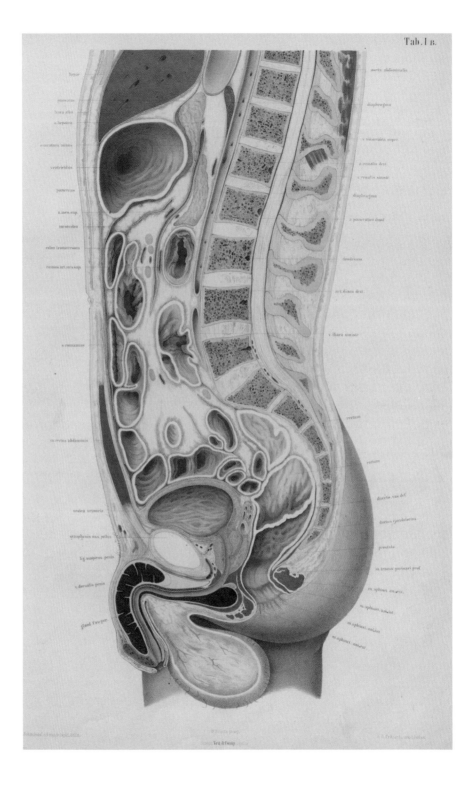

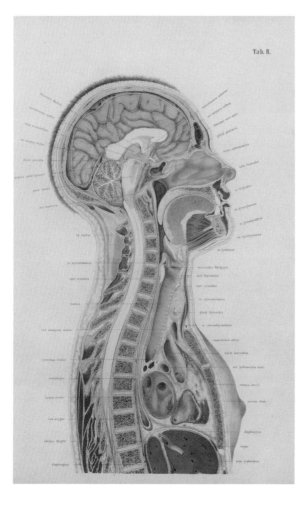

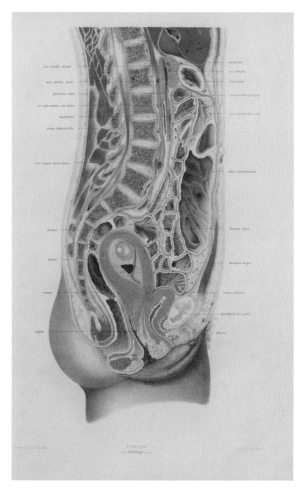

*Topographisch-anatomischer
Atlas* (1867)

Opposite: A section through
the abdomen of a male cadaver.
Above: A two-part image of
the head and body of a female
cadaver.

the body to extend the life, as it were, of the corpse. The practice spread from the anatomy theatre to the funeral shop as mourners, for sentimental reasons, wished to preserve the memory of their late loved one's appearance as long as possible. Undertakers were a nineteenth-century invention.

The combination of improved embalming techniques and the expansion of the railway system meant that the bereaved could honour the deceased's wishes to be buried in a favourite place far from the place of death. Embalming was widely used during the American Civil War (1861–5) to enable the return of the bodies of fallen soldiers to their homes and families.

The German chemist August Wilhelm von Hofmann discovered formaldehyde in 1869, which proved to have excellent preservative properties although, ironically, it was a skin irritant. Others found other ways. The Polish anatomist Zygmunt Laskowski (1841–1928) had success with a mixture of phenol and glycerine in 1866 (later replacing the glycerine with alcohol) and published two books on the subject: *Les procédés de conservation des pièces anatomiques* (*Conservation Procedures for Anatomical Specimens)* in 1885 and *L'embaumement et la conservation des sujets et des préparations anatomiques* (*Embalming and Conservation of Subjects and Anatomical Preparations*) the following year.

The sum of Laskowski's work was his *Anatomie normale du corps humain: atlas iconographique* (*Iconographic Atlas of the Normal Anatomy of the Human Body*), published in 1893 in Geneva, Laskowski's adopted home. It is a magnificent book with which to see the nineteenth century out. Its sixteen accurately printed colour plates were a model of diagrammatic clarity, each image showing only what was important and intended.

Under Laskowski's direction the very modern illustrations were drawn by Zygmunt Balicki (1858–1916), a fellow Pole in exile and a comrade in arms. Both men were members of the *Liga Narodowa* (National League), a secret organisation campaigning for political reform in their homeland, then very much a satellite of Tsarist Russia. Balicki was instrumental in its founding in 1893, the year of *Atlas iconographique*'s publication. Laskowski had been forced into exile in Paris after taking part in a failed uprising in Warsaw in 1863, while Balicki was deported to Switzerland in 1883 following his arrest as a leader of the Polish Socialist Commune.

Laskowski had been a field surgeon for French forces in the 1870 war with Prussia, which led to the establishment of the German Empire. Balicki, who studied art in St Petersburg, found his way into print in 1896 with *L'état comme organisation coercitive de la société politique* (*The State as a Coercive Organisation of Political Society*). He died of a heart condition in St Petersburg in 1916, having played a significant role there in the preparation of the Russian Revolution. The rise of the German Empire and the demise of the Russian one would be the defining political upheavals of the coming century.

Anatomy does not exist in a vacuum. Its progress is shaped by the cultures of the age, restricted at times by religious practice, advanced at others by the brutality of war and the repair of the wounded man, and at others by the technical innovations in its own and other fields. It is always, however, driven by scientists who allow themselves the luxury of curiosity and the courage of experimentation.

Often overlooked in the history of anatomy are the souls whose bodies were the anatomists' laboratories and without whom anatomy's progress was often curtailed. These were real people. Carl von Rokitansky (1804–78), the founder of the Viennese School of Medicine, whose three-volume *Handbuch der pathologischen Anatomie* (*Handbook of Pathological Anatomy*) was compulsory reading for all medical students in the Austro-Hungarian Empire after its publication in 1846, wrote compassionately in 1876:

> As you bend with the rigid blade of your scalpel over the unknown corpse, remember that this body was born of the love of two souls; it grew rocked by faith and for the hope of the one who sheltered him in her bosom. He smiled and dreamed the same dreams as children and young people. Certainly he loved and was loved, he hoped and cherished a happy tomorrow, and he missed the others who had departed. Now it lies on the cold slate, without a single tear having been shed for it, without a single prayer. His name, only God knows. But inexorable fate gave him the power and greatness to serve humanity.

Zygmundt Laskowski (1841–1928) preserved his specimens in a mixture of phenol and alcohol.

Hofmann discovered formaldehyde, an invaluable aid to the preservation of cadavers.

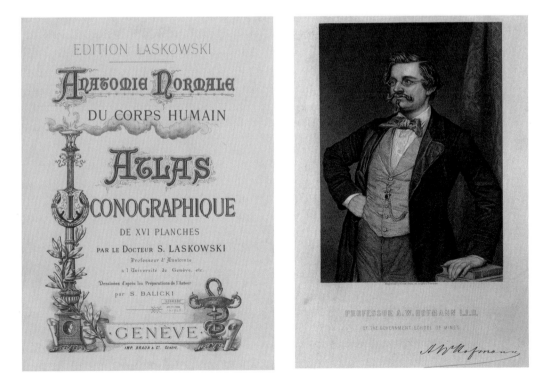

Atlas iconographique (1893)

Right: Fine studies of the spine and joints, drawn for Laskowski by Zygmunt Balicki (1858–1916). Opposite: Details of the teeth, throat, mouth and other viscera.

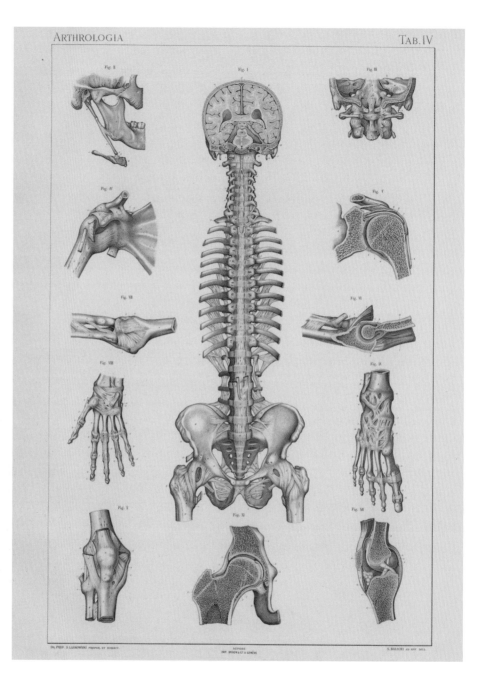

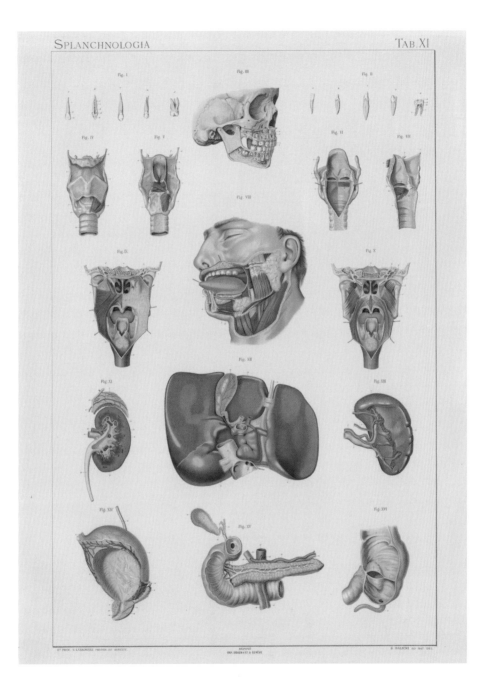

TAB. VIII

Atlas iconographique (1893)

Right: An overview of the muscles, pulmonary system and viscera of the torso. Opposite: Studies of the sense organs – eyes, nose, ears and mouth – and hair follicles.

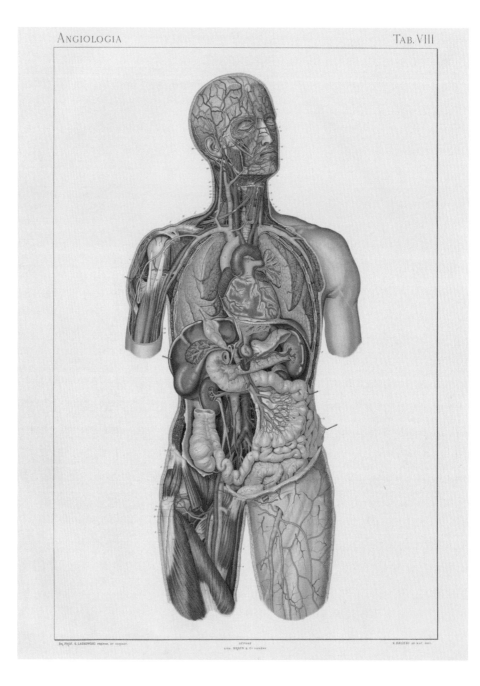

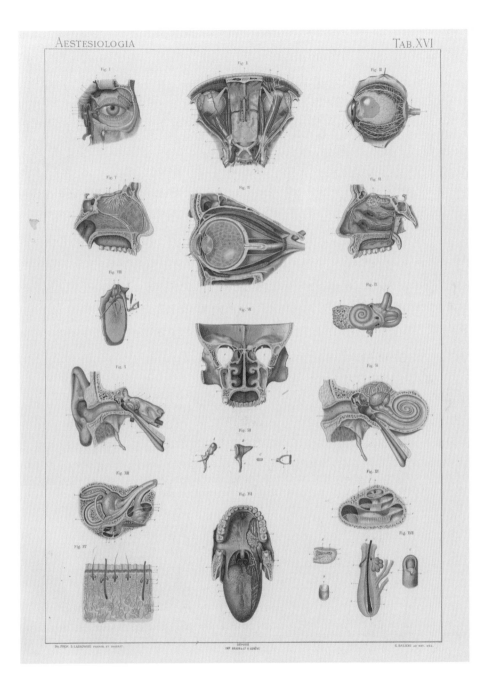

WHAT HAPPENED NEXT?

By the end of the nineteenth century the macroscopic understanding of human anatomy was more or less complete. There was a name for every part that one could see with the naked eye, and a good understanding of how all the parts functioned and interacted with each other. Myths had been dispelled. The study of anatomy was now, as far as anatomists from Ancient Egypt onwards had been trying to understand it, concluded.

Yet at the start of the twentieth century the quiet revolution begun by those eighteenth-century pioneers of the microscope was now the driving force behind medical research. A new age of anatomy was focussing on the cellular and sub-cellular components of the human body. These elements of human tissue, which could no longer be seen or understood by ordinary people, might have reduced the public's interest in the science or deepened its mistrust of anatomists. In practice, however, the opposite has been true. The steady march of technological progress in the twentieth and twenty-first centuries has made us all far more scientifically literate than our predecessors; and although we may not all understand everything we see, we take a scientific interest.

Making anatomy visible

The greatest technological advances of the last 120 years stem from Philipp Bozzini's *Lichtleiter* (light conductor), that first endoscope. The possibility of seeing inside a living body, unimaginable before 1817, was made real by Wilhelm Röntgen's discovery of X-rays in 1895. As the medical profession learned how to use this extraordinary new tool, one the first textbooks to accommodate it was Arthur Appleton, William Hamilton and Ivan Tchaperoff's *Surface and Radiological Anatomy*, published in 1938. Thirty years later Isadore Meschan explored the very practical question of how to get the best view of the desired area of the body, in his *Radiographic Positioning and Related Anatomy*.

X-rays are old-fashioned now, but only towards the end of the last century were more detailed imaging techniques developed. Now computer tomography (CT) scans and magnetic resonance imaging (MRI) are commonplace, and scanning electron microscopes are capable of three million times magnification and resolutions greater than a single nanometre (a billionth of a metre). Today the go-to manual is *Musculoskeletal MRI* by Clyde Helms, Nancy Major, Mark Anderson, Phoebe Kaplan and Robert Dussault. First published in 2008, its subject is a fast-evolving one and a third edition was already required in 2020.

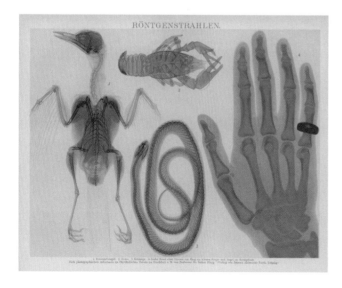

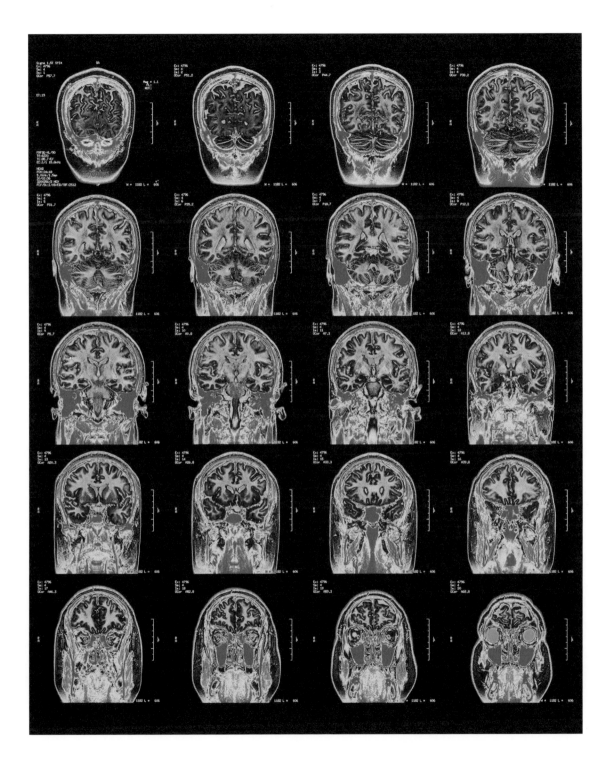

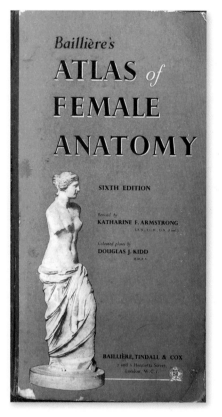

ABOVE

Baillière's Atlas of Female Anatomy (6th edition)

A rare example of an anatomy book devoted entirely to the female sex, its first edition appeared in 1942.

OPPOSITE

Topographische Anatomie des Menschen (1937)

The muscle layer next to the thoracic cage, from Eduard Pernkopf's brilliant but unethically derived Anatomy.

Publishing landmarks

Images produced with these devices routinely illustrate anatomy texts now, alongside traditional photography. Sometimes, however, a diagram is still the best way to instruct. New anatomies are still published from time to time, many hoping to carve out a piece of the student market still served by *Gray's Anatomy*. One long overdue volume made its debut in 1942 – Ballière's *Popular Atlas of the Anatomy and Physiology of the Female Human Body* by Hubert E.J. Biss, with illustrations by Georges Dupuy, perhaps the first publication devoted entirely to that gender. Baillière (later Baillière, Tindall and Cox) emerged as a leading anatomy publisher in the nineteenth century, and its *Atlas of Female Anatomy* was still in print in 1969, in its seventh edition.

The professionalisation of the role of nurses after the First World War opened a new market for anatomy authors and publishers. Ernest William Hey Groves and John Matthew Fortescue-Brickdale launched their four-volume *Text-book for Nurses* in 1921, addressing anatomy, physiology, surgery and medicine. Katharine Armstrong's *Aids to Anatomy and Physiology: Textbook for the Nurse* first appeared in 1939 and, like *Gray's Anatomy*, outlived its author, running to at least nine editions. Armstrong edited later editions of Baillière's *Atlas of Female Anatomy*; by the time her *Textbook for the Nurse* got into print, Evelyn Pearce's *Anatomy and Physiology for Nurses* (first published in 1929) was already in its fourth edition: its sixteenth arrived in 1975. Pearce was a prolific author for nurses and her *Medical and Nursing Dictionary and Encyclopaedia* of 1935 did for nurses what Sir Richard Quain's *Dictionary of Medicine* had done for doctors fifty years earlier.

One anatomy still used today is rarely discussed and, despite its excellence as a reference work, has been out of print since 1994. The book, Eduard Pernkopf's *Topographische Anatomie des Menschen* (*Pernkopf's Atlas of Topographic and Applied Anatomy of Man*), was first published in 1937 and, by reputation, contains the finest anatomical illustrations ever published. Some surgeons still rely on it for their work; but others find themselves unable to use it unless they are able to discuss its history with their patients first. Pernkopf, an Austrian, was an ardent support of Adolf Hitler and wore a Nazi uniform to work. He taught at the University of Vienna, where he dismissed all Jewish staff, including three Nobel laureates. The magnificent images in his four-volume masterpiece are of the bodies of those executed by the Nazi regime, which pursued an imagined racial purity by murdering homosexuals, gypsies, dissidents and Jews.

Pernkopf's Atlas raises the ethical question of whether a book resulting from such cruelty and death should be used to save lives. Pernkopf returned to the University of Vienna after the Second World War. The fourth volume was published just after his death in 1955 and the book was translated and widely published around the world. Only in the 1990s were questions asked about his wartime record. Leaders of the Jewish community are of the view that *Pernkopf's Atlas* can be used to do medical good, provided the truth about its images is made known.

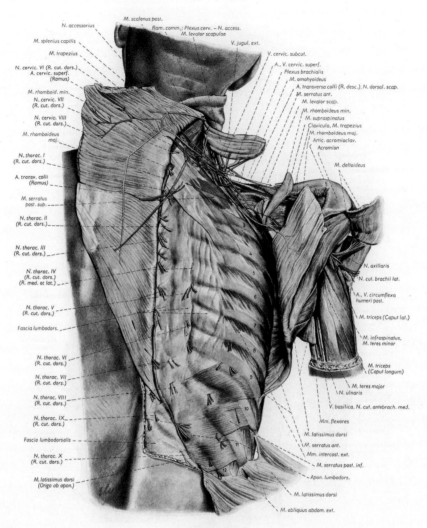

M. scalenus post.
N. accessorius
Ram. comm.; Plexus cerv. – N. access.
M. levator scapulae
M. splenius capitis
V. jugul. ext.
M. trapezius
V. cervic. subcut.
N. cervic. VI (R. cut. dors.)
A., V. cervic. superf.
A. cervic. superf.
Plexus brachialis
(Ramus)
M. omohyoideus
M. rhomboid. min.
A. transversa colli (R. desc.), N. dorsal. scap.
N. cervic. VII
M. serratus ant.
(R. cut. dors.)
M. levator scap.
M. rhomboideus min.
N. cervic. VIII
M. supraspinatus
(R. cut. dors.)
Clavicula, M. trapezius
M. rhomboideus
M. rhomboideus maj.
maj.
Artic. acromioclav.
Acromion
N. thorac. I
(R. cut. dors.)
A. transv. colli
M. deltoideus
(Ramus)
M. serratus
post. sup.
N. thorac. II
(R. cut. dors.)
N. thorac. III
(R. cut. dors.)
N. thorac. IV
(R. cut. dors.)
N. axillaris
(R. med. et lat.)
N. cut. brachii lat.
A., V. circumflexa
humeri post.
N. thorac. V
(R. cut. dors.)
M. triceps (Caput lat.)
Fascia lumbodors.
M. infraspinatus,
M. teres minor
N. thorac. VI
(R. cut. dors.)
N. thorac. VII
M. triceps
(R. cut. dors.)
(Caput longum)
N. thorac. VIII
M. teres major
(R. cut. dors.)
N. ulnaris
N. thorac. IX
V. basilica, N. cut. antebrach. med.
(R. cut. dors.)
Mm. flexores
Fascia lumbodorsalis
M. latissimus dorsi
M. serratus ant.
N. thorac. X
Mm. intercost. ext.
(R. cut. dors.)
M. serratus post. inf.
M. latissimus dorsi
Apon. lumbodors.
(Origo ab apon.)
M. latissimus dorsi
M. obliquus abdom. ext.

3–12 = ribs

Fig. 24. View of muscle layer which is in direct contact with the thoracic cage, after removal of the rhomboid and levator scapulae muscles, thus displacing the scapula anteriorly. Exposure of both serratus posterior muscles and the fascia of the intrinsic back muscles (lumbodorsal fascia).

Fig. 24

The supply of cadavers

Apart from the obvious benefits of modern scans for examination and diagnosis, they also reduce the anatomy lecturer's dependence on cadavers. Plaster and plastic anatomical teaching models have replaced some real body parts since the late eighteenth century; and now scans (whether live or reproduced in books) are central to the learning process.

In some cases, however, there is no substitute for a human being. At the University of Berkeley in the United States and other institutions, anatomy students are encouraged to palpate themselves or volunteers (the anatomy equivalent of an artists' models) to explore the surface of their own or other bodies for evidence of the anatomy within. Palpation is very old technique for diagnosis, commonly used before anaesthesia made exploratory surgery an option. At the University of Birmingham, England, the anatomy department (in order to reduce its dependence on cadavers) has returned to the sixteenth century practice of demonstration. Instead of dissecting several corpses, a whole cohort of students watches a prosector and dissector conduct and explain the dissection of a single body.

It's a return to the teaching practices which persisted for 400 years until the early nineteenth century. With the regulation introduced in that century, anatomy training was gradually absorbed into the university curriculum, where it was conducted behind closed doors, away from the public gaze.

Public fascination

The public, however, is still curious. Since the Second World War the publishing industry has recognised this with an increasing number of anatomy books aimed at lay readers – and their children. Ilse Goldsmith's *Anatomy for Children*, published in New York in 1964, was an early example. In the twenty-first century there are even anatomy colouring books for all ages, from Kelly Solloway's *The Yoga Anatomy Coloring Book* (2018), a meeting of anatomy and mindfulness, to *The Human Anatomy and Physiology Coloring Book* (2020) with its cartoon-like line drawings aimed at reassuring young patients.

Lay adults have been entertained by several landmark, factual medical series on television. The BBC broke new ground with *Your Life in Their Hands*, a long-running series about surgery, originally presented by Charles Fletcher from 1958 to 1964, then by Jonathan Miller in

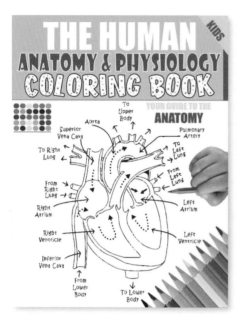

ABOVE

The Human Anatomy and Physiology Coloring Book (2020)

Anatomy books for children are evidence of society's changing attitudes to a subject which was once taboo.

RIGHT

Gunther von Hagens (b. 1945)

The showman-anatomist with his trademark black hat and a plastinated horse.

the early 1970s and by Robert Winston from 1979 to 1987. Miller also presented *The Body in Question*, a thirteen-part series, in 1978; and Winston went on to front many TV series including *The Human Body* in 1998.

One controversial aspect of the public's continuing interest in anatomy has been the work of Gunther von Hagens. Hagens devised a technique called plastination for preserving human tissue, at first in small samples and specimens and now whole human and animal bodies. He presents these in various stages of dissection in public exhibitions called *Body Worlds* (to date, there have been four *Body Worlds*). Human bodies can take up to 1,500 hours to plastinate; and a giraffe exhibited in *Body Worlds Three* took three years to preserve.

Hagens insists that the human bodies he exhibits are all donated willingly before their deaths, but some religious bodies have objected to the public display of bodies in this way. Many of the objections to his practice are the same ones which have always been levelled at anatomists – unproven accusations of buying corpses from body snatchers in Novosibirsk, or of using executed prisoners from China and Kyrgyzstan. In 2002 he performed an illegal public dissection in a packed London theatre which was subsequently broadcast on Britain's Channel 4 television network. Hagens was not prosecuted, but he may have found the limits of the appeal of anatomy to the mass market.

Hagens always wears a black fedora when conducting public autopsies, a reference to Rembrandt's painting *The Anatomy Lesson of Dr Nicolaes Tulp*. Anatomy continues to be an important part of an artist's training, and after losing some favour towards the end of the twentieth century it is enjoying a revival of interest in art schools. The twentieth century produced many books aimed at the artist, many of them privately published by fellow artists hoping to expand their income. Some artists are better than others, and two particularly fine American examples of the genre are Victor Perard's *Anatomy and Drawing* (1928) and Charles Carlson's *A Simplified Art Anatomy of the Human Figure* (1941). Both are still in print as facsimile editions today.

Anatomy as a metaphor

Anatomy, then, continues to fascinate. If there were any doubt, then one publishing fashion in the second half of the twentieth century should dispel it. An outrider for the trend, *The Anatomy of Peace*, was published in 1945. Its author Emery Reves was, among other things, Winston Churchill's literary agent, and his book argued for global federalism as a means of ensuring peace after the Second World War. But it was Robert Traver (the pen name of Michigan Supreme Court Justice John D. Voelker) who really made it fashionable. In 1958 he published his new novel, *Anatomy of a Murder*, a fictional version of a real-life murder trial over which he had presided in 1952. The film of the book, directed by Otto Preminger, starring James Stewart and scored by Duke Ellington, was a big hit on its release the following year.

What could not have been foreseen was the public fascination with the title. It was clever, evoking the dead body of the victim; but the metaphor of anatomy caught the

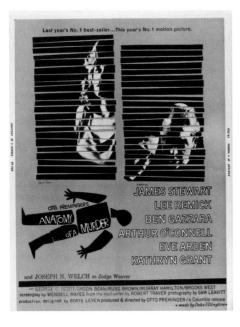

Anatomy of a Murder (1959)

A poster for Otto Preminger's film of Robert Traver's book, based on the murder trial in which Traver was the defence attorney. In the mid-twentieth century anatomy was a popular metaphor for close examination of any kind.

imagination of readers and writers for more than a decade afterwards. Book after book was published whose titles all began 'Anatomy of a . . .'. Many of them were in the sensational tradition of pulp fiction or 'true crime': *Anatomy of a Psycho* by Alex M. Szedenik (1964); Gary Gordon's *The Anatomy of Adultery, with Case Histories* (1964); and King Coral's *The Anatomy and the Ecstasy* (1966), to name but three.

There were also attempts to write popular books on serious subjects: Ladislas Farago's *War of Wits: The Anatomy of Espionage and Intelligence* (1954); Cornel Lengyel's *I, Benedict Arnold: The Anatomy of Treason* (1960), a biography of an American officer during America's War of Independence who defected to the British Army; and *Anatomy of Automation* (1962), George and Paul Amber's thoughtful history of robotics, to name another three.

The craze for *Anatomy* titles petered out in the late 1960s, but new ones still appear occasionally. They may seem irrelevant in an anatomist's library; but collectively they fixed anatomy, whether as metaphor or as study of the structures of the body, firmly in the mind of the public. Robert Traver – who was neither a murderer nor an anatomist – quit the law courts on the strength of the success of *Anatomy of a Murder*. In retirement he was a keen angler and wrote three popular fishing memoirs, including (in 1964 at the height of the craze he had started) *Anatomy of a Fisherman*.

Anatomy of the brain

Current research is using detailed imaging techniques to chart the evolutionary processes which have shaped our anatomy. Pathological anatomy faces increasingly frequent challenges from viral epidemics such as bovine spongiform encephalopathy (BSE), severe acute respiratory syndrome (SARS) and other strains of coronavirus. Advances in molecular biology are helping us to understand the functions of our organs; and as physicists unravel the subatomic mysteries of the universe, their discoveries will no doubt lead to paradigm shifts in anatomy in the coming decades.

Those future breakthroughs are for another book. This one celebrates the landmarks of the past, and the great anatomists who erected them in picture and print, filling a whole library with their work. Modern instruments have revolutionised the visibility of anatomy; but it's worth noting that understanding what is visible remains the task, as it has been for thousands of years, of the remarkable human brain. So far at least, that is irreplaceable.

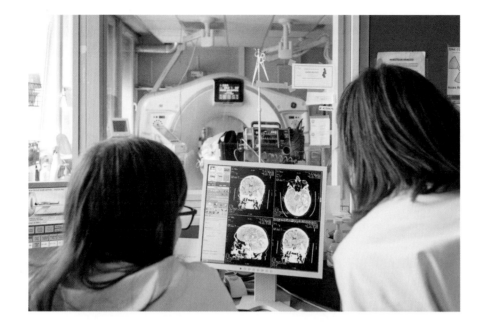

LEFT

CT scans

Above: Medical technicians examine a patient's head non-invasively through images generated by computerised tomography. Below: A patient undergoing a CT scan. New technology gives us unparalleled views of the workings of the human body; but understanding what it sees is still the work of the extraordinary human brain.

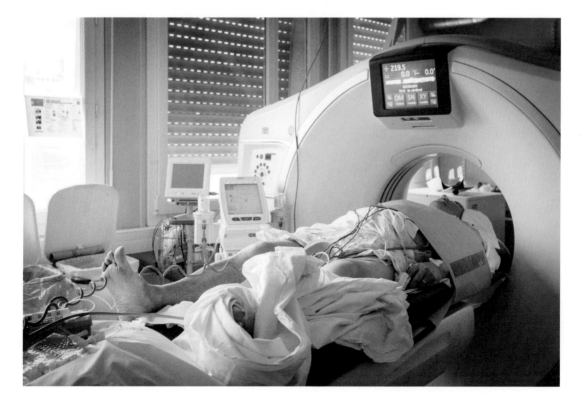

BIBLIOGRAPHY

Chapter 1: Anatomy in the Ancient World

*c.*3000 BCE, Unknown, Edwin Smith Papyrus, Egypt

*c.*3000 BCE, Unknown, Georg Ebers Papyrus, Egypt

*c.*2000 BCE, Unknown, Brugsch Papyrus, Egypt

*c.*1800 BCE, Unknown, Kahun Papyrus, Egypt

*c.*1800 BCE, Unknown, Hearst Papyrus, Egypt

*c.*550 BCE, Alcmaeon, *On Nature*, Greece

*c.*450–150 BCE, Unknown, *Huangdi Neijing*, China

*c.*400–370 BCE, Hippocrates, The Hippocratic Corpus, Greece

*c.*300–280 BCE, Herophilos, On Pulses, Greece

*c.*300–280 BCE, Herophilos, Midwifery, Greece

*c.*200 CE, Galen, *On Anatomical Procedures*, Rome

*c.*200 CE, Galen, *On the Functions of the Different Parts of the Human Body*, Rome

*c.*200 CE, Galen, *On Semen*, Rome

*c.*200 CE, Galen, *On Foetal Formation*, Rome

*c.*200 CE, Galen, *On the Dissection of the Uterus*, Rome

*c.*200 CE, Galen, *Is Blood Naturally Contained in the Arteries?*, Rome

c. 200 CE, Galen, *On My Own Books*, Rome

*c.*860, Hunayn ibn Ishāq (translator), *On Bones for Beginners*, Baghdad

*c.*860, Hunayn ibn Ishāq (translator), *On Anatomical Procedures*, Baghdad

*c.*860, Hunain ibn Ishāq, *Ten Treatises of the Eye*, Baghdad

*c.*900, Rhazes, *Doubts about Galen*, Tehran

*c.*900, Rhazes, *For One Who Has No Physician to Attend Him*, Tehran

c. 940, Rhazes, *The Virtuous Life*, Tehran

1025, Avicenna, *The Canon of Medicine*, Tehran

1288, Ibn al-Nafis, *The Comprehensive Book on Medicine*, Egypt

1316 (published 1475), Mondino de Luzzi, *The Anatomy of the Human Body*, Bologna

Chapter 2: Medieval Anatomy

*c.*1120, Zayn al-Din al-Jurjani, *Thesaurus of the Shah of Khwarazm*, Persia

*c.*1335, Guido da Vigevano, *Health Manual*, France

1345, Guido da Vigevano, *An Anatomy for Philippe VII*, France

1390, Mansur ibn Ilyas, *Anatomy of the Human Body*, Shiraz

1491, Johannes de Ketham (compiler), *Medical Anthology*, Venice

1497, Hieronymus Brunschwig, *The Book of Surgery*

1499, Johann Peyligk, *Compendium of Natural Philosophy*, Leipzig

1501, Magnus Hundt, *Anthropology of the Dignity of Man, Nature and Properties, of the Elements, Parts and Members of the Human Body*, Leipzig

1503, Gregor Reisch, *A Philosophical Pearl*, Strasbourg

1507, Antonio Benivieni, *The Hidden Causes of Disease*, Florence

1512, Hieronymus Brunschwig, *Book of the Art of Compound Distilling*, Strasbourg

1516–24, Alessandro Achillini, *Anatomy of the Human Body*, Venice

1520, Alessandro Achillini, *Anatomical Notes*, Bologna

Chapter 3: Anatomy in the Renaissance

*c.*30 BCE, Vitruvius, *On Architecture*, Rome

1517, Hans von Gersdorff, *Field Book of Surgery*, Strasbourg

1522, Jacopo Berengario da Carpi, *A Brief Introduction . . . to the Anatomy of the Human Body*, Bologna

1528, Albrecht Dürer, *Four Books on Human Proportion*, Nuremberg

1539, Jean Ruel (compiler), *Veterinary Medicine*, Paris

1538, Heinrich Vogtherr, *Anatomy*, Strasbourg

1543, Andreas Vesalius, *On the Fabric of the Human Body in Seven Books*, Basel

1544, Jacob Frölich, *Anatomy*, Strasbourg

1545, Charles Estienne, *On the Dissection of the Parts of the Human Body, in Three Books*, Paris

1545, Ambroise Paré, *The Method of Curing Wounds Caused by Arquebus and Firearms*

1551, Conrad Gessner, *History of Animals*, Zurich

1552 , Juan Valverde de Amusco, *A Pamphlet on the Preservation of Mental and Physical Health*, Paris

1556, Juan Valverde de Amusco, *History of the Composition of the Human Body*, Rome

1559, Realdo Colombo, *Fifteen Books about Anatomy*

1561, Gabriele Falloppio, *Anatomical Observations*, Venice

1575, Ambroise Paré, *Collected Works*, Paris

1598, Carlo Ruini, *Anatomy of the Horse*, Venice

1714, Bartholomeo Eustachi, *Anatomical Charts*, Rome

1898, Leonardo da Vinci, *Leonardo da Vinci's Manuscripts from the Royal Library of Windsor: On Anatomy*, Paris

Chapter 4: The Age of the Microscope

1553, Miguel Servet, *The Restoration of Christianity*

1595, Jehan Cousin the Younger, *Book of Portraiture*, Paris

1600, Girolamo Fabrici, *On the Formed Foetus*, Frankfurt

1601, Giulio Casseri, *The Anatomical History of the Voice and Organs of Hearing*

1603, Girolamo Fabrici, *On the Speech of Animals*

1603, Girolamo Fabrici, *On Speech and its Instruments*

1613, Girolamo Fabrici, *Triple Anatomical Treatise*

1613, Johann Remmelin, *A Mirror of the Microcosm*, Augsburg

1621, Girolamo Fabrici, *On the Formation of the Egg and the Chicken*

1626, Adriaan van Spiegel and Giulio Casseri, *On the Formed Foetus*, Padua

1627, Adriaan van Spiegel and Giulio Casseri, *Anatomical Charts*, Venice

1628, William Harvey, *An Anatomical Account of the Motion of the Heart and Blood*, Frankfurt

1644, Giovanni Battista Hodierna, *The Eye of the Fly*, Palermo

1648, William Molins, *Myskotomia, or The Anatomical Administration of all the Muscles of an Humane Body*

1661, Marcello Malpighi, *Anatomical Observations of the Lungs*, Bologna

1664, Thomas Willis, *The Anatomy of the Brain*

1665, Robert Hooke, *Micrographia*, London

1666, Marcello Malpighi, *The Polyp in the Heart*

1668, Reinier de Graaf, *On the Organs of Men which Serve for Generation*

1672, Thomas Willis, *Two Discourses concerning the Soul of Brutes, which is that of the Vital and Sensitive of Man*

1672, Jan Swammerdam and Johannes van Horne, *A Miracle of Nature or the Device of a Woman's Womb*

1672, Reinier de Graaf, *A new Treatise on the Organs of Women which Serve for Generation*

1675, Marcello Malpighi, *Anatomy of the Plants*

1676, Charles Scarborough, *Syllabus of the Muscles*, Oxford

1678, John Browne, *A Compleat Discourse of Wounds*

1681, John Browne, *A Compleat Treatise of the Muscles*, London

1683, Andrew Snape, *The Anatomy of an Horse*

1684, Raymond Vieussens, *A Complete Neurology*, Paris

1685, Govard Bidloo, *Anatomy of the Human Body*, Amsterdam

1694, William Cowper, *Myotomia Reformata, or a New Administration of the Muscles*

1695, Humphrey Ridley, *The Anatomy of the Brain, containing its Mechanism and Physiology*, London

1697, Edward Ravenscroft, *The Anatomist, or The Sham-Doctor*

1698, William Cowper, *The Anatomy of Humane Bodies*, Oxford

1705, Raymond Vieussens, *A New Vascular System of the Human Body*

1737, Jan Swammerdam, *Bible of Nature*, Leiden

Chapter 5: The Age of Enlightenment

1304, Shozen Kajiwara, *Book of the Simple Physician*

1679, Théophile Bonet, *The Cemetery, or Anatomy Practiced from Corpses Dead of Disease*

1706–19, Giovanni Battista Morgagni, *Anatomical Adversaries*

1713, William Cheselden, *The Anatomy of the Humane Body*

1731, Jacques-François-Marie Duverney, *Treatise on the Organ of Hearing*

1733, William Cheselden, *Osteographia, or The Anatomy of the Bones*, London

1735, Antonio Maria Valsalva, *A Treatise on the Human Ear*

1743, William Hunter, *On the Structure and Diseases of Articulating Cartilages*

1746, Jacques Fabien Gautier d'Agoty and Jacques-François-Marie Duverney, *Complete Myology in Colour and Natural Size*, Paris

1747, Bernhard Seigfried Albinus, *Diagrams of the Skeleton and Muscles of the Human Body*, London

1748, Jacques Fabien Gautier d'Agoty and Jacques-François-Marie Duverney, *Anatomy of the Head*, Paris

1749, Jacques-François-Marie Duverney, *The Art of Methodically Dissecting the Muscles of the Human Body, Made Accessible to Beginners*

1752, Jacques Fabian Gautier d'Agoty, *General Anatomy of the Viscera in Situation: of Natural Size and Colour*, Paris

1754, William Smellie, *A Sett of Anatomical Tables*, London

1752–1764, William Smellie, *A Treatise on the Theory and Practice of Midwifery*

1759, Tōyō Yamawaki, *Notes on the Viscera*

1761, Giovani Battista Morgagni, *Of the Seats and Causes of Diseases Investigated through Anatomy*

1772, Kawaguchi Shinnin, *Analysis of Cadavers*, Heian [Kyoto]

1774, William Hunter, *The Anatomy of the Human Gravid Uterus Exhibited in Figures*, Birmingham, England

1774, Johann Adam Kulmus, Gempaku Sugita, Ryotaku Maeno, Junnan Nakagawa and Hoshu Katsuragawa, *A New Book of Anatomy*, Tokyo

1998, Hilary Mantel, *The Giant*, O'Brien

Chapter 6: The Age of Invention

1789, Antonio Scarpa, *Anatomical Investigations of Hearing and Smell*

1794, Antonio Scarpa, *Neurological Records*

1795, Samuel Thomas von Sömmerring, *A Chart of the Female Skeleton*, Frankfurt

1800, Xavier Bichat, *Treatise on Membranes*

1800, Xavier Bichat, *Physiological Researches upon Life and Death*

1801, Xavier Bichat, *General Anatomy*

1801, Samuel Thomas von Sömmerring, *Pictures of the Human Eye*

1801, Antonio Scarpa, *A Treatise on the Principal Diseases of the Eyes*

1801–1814, Leopoldo Marco Antonio Caldani, *Anatomical Images*, Venice

1805, Hanaoka Seishū, *Findings on Breast Cancer*

1806, Samuel Thomas von Sömmerring, *Pictures of the Human Ear*

1806, Samuel Thomas von Sömmerring, *Pictures of the Human Organ of Taste and Voice*

1807, Philipp Bozzini, *The Light Conductor . . . for Illuminating Inner Cavities and Interstices of the Living Animal Body*

1809, Samuel Thomas von Sömmerring, *Pictures of the Human Organ of Smell*

1809, Franz Joseph Gall and Johann Gaspar Spurzheim, *Investigations into the Anatomy of the Nervous System in General, and of the Brain in Particular*

1819, Franz Joseph Gall, *The Anatomy and Physiology of the Nervous System . . .*

1828, Jones Quain, *Elements of Descriptive and Practical Anatomy for the Use of Students*

1829, John MacNee, *The Trial of William Burke and Helen M'Dougal*

1830, Domenico Cotugno, *Posthumous Works*

1832, Joseph Vimont, *Treatise of Human and Comparative Phrenology*, Paris

1837, Hanaoka Seishū, *Surgical Casebook*

1844, Richard Quain, *The Anatomy of the Arteries of the Human Body*, London

1846, Carl von Rokitansky, *Handbook of Pathological Anatomy*

1858, Henry Gray, *Anatomy: Descriptive and Surgical* (*Gray's Anatomy*)

1858, Rudolph Virchow, *Cellular Pathology*

1859, Charles Darwin, *On the Origin of Species*

1861, Pierre Paul Broca, *Remarks on the Seat of the Function of Spoken Language*

1867, Christian Wilhelm Braune, *Topographical Anatomy Atlas: from Cross-Sections of Frozen Cadavers,* Leipzig
1873, Christian Wilhelm Braune, *The Position of the Uterus and Foetus at the End of Pregnancy from Cross-Sections of Frozen Cadavers*
1882, Sir Richard Quain, *Quain's Dictionary of Medicine*
1885, Zygmunt Laskowski, *Conservation Procedures for Anatomical Specimens*
1886, Zygmunt Laskowski, *Embalming and Conservation of Subjects and Anatomical Preparations*
1893, Zygmunt Laskowski, *Iconographic Atlas of the Normal Anatomy of the Human Body,* Geneva
1931, James Bridie, *The Anatomist*
1966, Sawako Ariyoshi, *The Doctor's Wife*

Postscript: What Happened Next

1921, Ernest William Hey Groves and John Matthew Fortescue-Brickdale, *Text-book for Nurses,* London
1928, Victor Perard, *Anatomy and Drawing,* USA
1929, Evelyn Pearce, *Anatomy and Physiology for Nurses,* London
1935, Evelyn Pearce, *Medical and Nursing Dictionary and Encyclopaedia,* London
1937, Eduard Pernkopf, *Pernkopf's Atlas of Topographic and Applied Anatomy of Man*
1938, Arthur Appleton, William Hamilton and Ivan Tchaperoff, *Surface and Radiological Anatomy,* Cambridge
1939, Katharine Armstrong, *Aids to Anatomy and Physiology: Textbook for the Nurse,* London
1941, Charles Carlson, *A Simplified Art Anatomy of the Human Figure,* New York
1942, (anonymous), *Baillière's Atlas of Female Anatomy,* London
1945, Emery Reves, *The Anatomy of Peace*
1954, Ladislas Farago, *War of Wits: The Anatomy of Espionage and Intelligence,* USA
1958, Robert Traver, *Anatomy of a Murder*
1960, Cornel Lengyel, I, Benedict Arnold: *The Anatomy of Treason*
1962, George and Paul Amber, *Anatomy of Automation,* Detroit
1964, Ilse Goldsmith, *Anatomy for Children,* New York
1964, Alex M. Szedenik, *Anatomy of a Psycho*
1964, Gary Gordon, *The Anatomy of Adultery, with Case Histories,* USA
1964, Robert Traver, *Anatomy of a Fisherman*
1966, King Coral, *The Anatomy and the Ecstasy*
1968, Isadore Meschan, *Radiographic Positioning and Related Anatomy*
1978, Jonathan Miller, *The Body in Question,* London
2008, Clyde Helms, Nancy Major, Mark Anderson, Phoebe Kaplan and Robert Dussault, *Musculoskeletal MRI*
2018, Kelly Solloway, *The Yoga Anatomy Coloring Book*
2020, (anonymous), *The Human Anatomy and Physiology Coloring Book*

INDEX

PICTURE CREDITS

The publishers thank the following for permission to reproduce the illustrations in this book. Every effort has been made to provide correct attributions. Any inadvertent errors or omissions will be corrected in subsequent editions.

(GraphicaArtis), 89 below left (DEA PICTURE LIBRARY), 91 (GraphicaArtis) , 92 (GraphicaArtis), 98 (Franco Origlia/Stringer), 100 (Leemage), 101 (GraphicaArtis), 156 above left (Universal History Archive), 157 (Science & Society Picture Library), 179 left (Science & Society Picture Library), 185 (Christophel Fine Art), 230 above (Stefano Bianchetti), 240 left below (Bettmann), 252 (mikroman6), 253 (Science Photo Library), 256–7 (Ted Soqui), 258 (LMPC), 259 above + below (BSIP)

Getty Research Institute: 108 left + right, 109, 110

Library of Congress: 65, 66, 67, 68

Metropolitan Museum of Art: 63, 94, 130, 131, 132 left + right

National Library of Medicine: 2, 41, 69 left + right, 70 above left, above right, below left + below right, 80, 81, 82 above left, above right, below left + below right, 96 above left, above right, below left + below right, 112 above + below, 113 left + right, 114 left + right, 115, 116 left + right, 117, 119, 120, 121 left, 122, 125 above left, above right + below, 126 left + right, 127 left + right, 134, 144 left + right, 145, 182, 183 above left, above right, below left + below right, 186, 187, 188 left + right, 189, 191, 192, 203, 204, 205, 206, 207, 208, 209 left + right, 213, 214, 215, 233, 234, 243 left + right, 244, 245 left + right, 247 left, 248, 249, 250, 251

Private Collection: 254, 255

Surgeons' Hall Museums, The Royal College of Surgeons of Edinburgh: 223

Wellcome Collection: 19, 20, 21, 24, 30 middle + right, 31, 32, 33, 44, 53 above left, above right, below left + below right, 60, 118, 124, 139, 147, 153, 154 left + right, 155 above left, above right + below, 156 above right + below, 164 left + right, 165 left, right above + right below, 165 right above + right below, 166 left + right, 167, 177 right, 190 above, 194 left above, left below + right, 195 left + right, 196, 197, 201 above, 216–17, 218 above, below left + below right, 220 left + right, 230 below, 231, 236 left + right, 237 left + right, 238, 239 left + right, 240 below, 247 right

Wikimedia Commons: 16, 47 (Biblioteca europea di informazione e cultura), 83 (National Gallery), 97 (Luc Viatour), 121 right (Biblioteca europea di informazione e cultura), 148 (Mauritshuis), 158 (Rijksmuseum)

ABOUT THE AUTHOR

Colin Salter is a science and history author and bibliophile living in Edinburgh, Scotland. He has written the *Science is Beautiful* trilogy (Batsford Books), a collection of micrographs of botany and the human body. He is the lead author of Pavilion Books' '100s' series, which includes *100 Books*, *100 Symbols* and *100 Science Discoveries that Changed the World*. His book *The Moon Landings* (Flame Tree Publishing) celebrated the fiftieth anniversary of the first man on the Moon. He has contributed to guidebooks on seashells, leaves and birdwatching, and with Michael Heatley he was co-author of *Everything You Wanted to Know about Inventions*. He has also written extensively about travel and popular music. He is currently writing *In My Father's Good Books*, the history of a 300-year-old library and the seven generations of the family which amassed it.

www.colinsalter.co.uk